Love in the Time of Forgetting

Love *in the* Time *of* Forgetting

A Memoir of Love and Life After Loss
with Lewy Body Dementia

BY Juanita Johnson

RESOURCE *Publications* · Eugene, Oregon

LOVE IN THE TIME OF FORGETTING
A Memoir of Love and Life After Loss with Lewy Body Dementia

Resource Publications
An Imprint of Wipf and Stock Publishers
199 W. 8th Ave., Suite 3
Eugene, OR 97401

www.wipfandstock.com

PAPERBACK ISBN: 979-8-3852-6183-3
HARDCOVER ISBN: 979-8-3852-6184-0
EBOOK ISBN: 979-8-3852-6185-7

VERSION NUMBER 01/15/26

For Earl, whose hand I held through both
remembering and forgetting.

And for every heart that has kept company
with memory's slow departure.

Contents

The Late Stage: February–May 2021

The Aftermath: Grief

CONTENTS

Acknowledgments

Collating these correspondences and journal entries into one place has been an act of love and of remembering. Though much of this journey was mine alone, I was not without help. I wish to express my gratitude to the following people:

First, to my daughter, Jen, for being my clear-sighted editor, pushing me hard to bring grit as well as grace to these pages. It was not an easy task for her to revisit her own grief as well as her mother's, yet she did so with courage and unwavering honesty. She reminded me again and again that truth has many textures—that love and loss, tenderness and pain, can live side by side in a single sentence. Her insight helped me find the balance between sorrow and strength, and her steady guidance shaped this story into its full and honest form. This book carries her imprint as surely as it carries mine.

And to my son, Rich, who was the first to read the manuscript, and whose many tears fell across its pages. His response—"We are some lucky-ass kids to have had our parents"—told me everything I needed to know about what endures. In his words, I heard the quiet truth of what our family has shared and the grace that continues to flow from it. His willingness to feel the full weight of this story reminded me that love, even when tested by loss, leaves behind a lasting legacy.

To Noah, my son-in-law, whose steady love was a quiet anchor through these years. His presence, so often expressed through simple gestures and a steadfast heart, reminded me that love doesn't always need words.

To my grandson, Sam, who kneaded dough beside me, sharing the quiet ritual of baking bread. Those simple acts became sacred time, binding us through touch, laughter, and the rhythm of doing something together. He showed a depth of love and compassion beyond his years.

To the friends who walked with me through the long seasons of illness, loss, and grief—and to those who may not be named in these pages but whose texts, emails, cards, kindness, and quiet companionship sustained me—thank you.

And to those who, in the years since Earl's death, have shared with me your own stories of caring for someone with Lewy body—your voices became companions as I wrote, lending me resolve and strength as this manuscript took shape.

Finally, to my publisher, who believed this story needed to be told and carried it forward with care and commitment. Thank you for helping it find its place in the world.

A Note from the Author

"You're navigating Lewy body dementia with love and intention. I wish there was a way you could share with others the way you and Earl are doing this."

I heard versions of this notion from several of the professionals Earl and I met with during his years living with Lewy body dementia (LBD). I took their words to heart. I hoped one day to write the story of our experience.

Before I share our story, I want to emphasize how strongly I believe luck is involved, especially as a factor determining which part of the brain is affected with cognitive decline. We were fortunate that Earl's brain allowed him to be gentle and kind most of the time. This isn't true for everyone. Would I have been able to care for Earl in the same ways if his disease caused him to be angry and resentful? I don't know. It would certainly have been much, much more difficult.

I also believe Earl's meditation practice and his extensive experiences with spiritual groups made his last years easier. I know his unflinching belief in love and forgiveness allowed him to accept his diagnosis and decline with grace. Earl had already let go of his grudges or unfinished business. He had focused on forgiveness for over a decade. His spiritual growth also allowed for honesty. The two of us talked often about how his body and mind were changing, and how those changes affected both of us. And it meant he did not fear dying. We openly talked about death, his and mine.

When Earl was diagnosed with Lewy body dementia in the spring of 2019, after several years of noting increasingly worrisome symptoms, I began writing in a new journal and sending email updates to family and friends. It was a way to carry on. Writing offered me the opportunity to clarify my feelings, feel connected, and receive comfort.

In the pages that follow, I hope you find something that can help you cope. I hope our experience can make your journey a bit easier, a bit less frightening, a bit less lonely.

May you find comfort and friendship in these pages.

The Prelude: September 2018–February 2019

September 14, 2018

Dear Present and Former Students,

I am writing to inform you I must stop offering classes, both in my home and through the Osher Lifelong Learning Institute (OLLI) at Duke.

As we all know, life has many twists and turns. My life has slowed to a crawl in order to be fully present with my husband of fifty-two years, who is declining. In slowing down, I hope to allow myself to feel all the losses, learn new lessons, grow in patience, breathe deeply, and know that the center will hold. The center will hold because the center is the great heart.

I'm aware of the importance of rallying support for both me and my husband. I have reached out to friends and suggested specific ways they can be supportive. I would encourage you to do the same, when a crisis arises in your life.

Feel gratitude for the blessings of your life. See them. Feel them.

In gratitude for each of you,
Juanita

Note: I sent this first correspondence, an email, to students of the classes I offered at OLLI and privately in my home—courses like "Aging with Grace," "Navigating Relationships with Adult Children," and "Writing an Ethical Will." I was increasingly aware that Earl was declining cognitively and physically. Earl was experiencing anxiety and emotional discomfort when I convened classes. He needed my full attention. After talking with family and friends, and doing some online research, I had a strong suspicion that Earl had Lewy body dementia. I knew I would miss my students and teaching, but I am grateful I had the financial means to be able to step back from this work.

January 24, 2019

Dear Mr. K, PA-C,

My husband, Earl S. Johnson, a patient of yours, is cognitively declining. He has an appointment with you on February 21, 2019. He also needs to be evaluated as soon as possible by someone who specializes in dementia.

Here are Earl's symptoms:

- Rapid breathing when climbing even a gentle hill
- Has fallen twice since his last appointment: in the shower and missing a stair step
- Hands shake
- Confusion. Some days are worse than others
- Agitation when confused or upset
- Sometimes can't finish a sentence
- Worrying, anxiety
- Shouting in middle of night, is scared or anxious
- Vivid dreams and sleep disturbances
- Twitching in his sleep
- Can't follow more than one-step directions; loses track or gets lost
- Hears a radio when no one else does; bothered by noises
- No sense of smell

These behaviors led me to do extensive research on cognitive deficits and decline. Given the research I have done, I think it is possible my brilliant husband has Lewy body dementia.

I appreciate the relationship you have with Earl. I know you will carefully evaluate his symptoms and proceed accordingly.

Sincerely,
Juanita Johnson

Note: This second correspondence was a letter to Earl's primary healthcare provider, a physician assistant who Earl saw through Veterans Affairs (VA). I sent this letter in advance of an appointment because I had read that, on average, a person with Lewy body dementia sees no fewer than eleven medical professionals before receiving a correct diagnosis.[1] I didn't want Earl (and I) to have to go through that. I wanted to be proactive. I was determined to be the best advocate I could be for my husband.

---

1. Snyder, *Treasures in the Darkness*, 24.

February 16, 2019

A few days ago, our daughter Jen, Earl, and I were sitting in our living room, talking about his upcoming appointment with his primary healthcare provider, and how we were seeking a diagnosis of Lewy body dementia. Earl became very angry. He verbally lashed out at Jen and me.

We both thought, "Oh God, is this what we are in store for?" If it is, am I up to the challenge?

Earl didn't seem to like me very much. He said, "The only way I will go to this appointment is if Jen takes me." I was being dismissed.

The incident scared both Jen and me. Earl was hostile and antagonistic.

Later that evening, a rash broke out on Earl's thigh. I asked our son-in-law Noah, a physician assistant who practices family medicine, to take a look. Noah said it looked like shingles. No wonder Earl had been so out of sorts.

I take this as a valuable lesson that, in someone with dementia, an infection can bring out disagreeable, ornery symptoms. The next day, after Earl was officially diagnosed and treated for shingles, his belligerent behavior stopped. A huge relief for all of us.

The Beginning: March 2019– December 2019

Daily Rhythms of Care

Our mornings begin quietly. I'm usually showered and dressed by 7:30 AM, moving through the morning with hushed intention.

By 8:00 AM, Earl begins to stir. He wakes slowly, sometimes with confusion, usually with tenderness. I greet him gently, help him orient to the time, what day it is, where he is.

"Good morning, Early Bird. It's morning now. You had a good night's sleep. It's a beautiful day. It's spring in North Carolina. We're home. We live next door to Jen Pooh, Noah, and Sam. Rich is safe and well, still sleeping until the sun rises on his home in Oregon." Earl nods, taking this in.

While Earl uses the bathroom, I lay out his clothes. He can dress himself, with a little help. Choosing clothes is the hardest part of dressing; it causes him stress and confusion. So, I choose for him.

By 9:00 AM, we're at the dining-room table. Breakfast is a diced orange and cereal or oatmeal. Afterward, he moves to the couch. He reads from a meditation book or fidgets with the iPad, looking for sudoku puzzles. I let these hours stretch, unhurried.

At noon, we share lunch. I've learned the rhythm of his appetite and have adjusted accordingly. A simple sandwich and some fruit he can pick up with his fingers are his favorites.

At 1:00 PM, a friend or family member arrives, so I can slip out for a walk or a trip to the grocery store. This hour away from the house is my daily chance to exhale. I have to be intentional about remembering this.

By 2:00 PM, Earl and I are side by side again, curled on our L-shaped couch. He naps; sometimes I nap, sometimes I read. He likes my sock feet in his lap. He rubs my feet until he nods off; this soothes him, and me. I've come to treasure this idiosyncratic, intimate ritual.

At 3:30 PM, if the weather is kind, we sit on our front porch. If not, we put on music from the 1960's and sway slowly together in the kitchen. Sometimes we dance. We are always close.

Earl likes to take a shower around 4:00 PM, and I do my best to make it a calming experience rather than a chore. It is clear to me from the way Earl becomes stressed and anxious if I seem rushed, that showering is a time I need to show a lot of gentleness and patience.

Supper follows, between 5:00 and 6:00 PM. Then a quiet hour of television, sitting on the couch, holding hands.

At 8:00 PM, we move through the bedtime routine: bathroom, brushing teeth, pajamas.

By 8:30 PM, I tuck him gently into bed, place a book in my lap, and read aloud to him, a few pages each evening. *Old Turtle*[1] is a favorite right now. After I read, we finish our nightly ritual with a breathing meditation, slowly breathing in and out together.

By 9:00 PM, he is asleep. I sit beside him for a moment before I kiss his cheek and whisper, "I'll see you in the morning light."

When Earl needs a medical appointment, I schedule it with care. Afternoons are best. He wants no unnecessary therapies and I honor that.

A medication calendar on the fridge makes it easy for me to keep track of meds. He never refuses his medications, which is a huge relief. Occasionally, Earl will ask what a medicine is and why he is taking it. I always tell him. He seems to trust my answers.

---

1. Wood, *Old Turtle*.

March 14, 2019

Dear Friends and Family,

Here begins my first update on our life with Lewy.

Two weeks ago, Earl's primary healthcare provider, Mr. K, examined Earl. At Earl's request, I was also present. Many of the questions Mr. K asked Earl were relevant to the letter I sent in advance of this appointment. In the letter, I had listed Earl's symptoms. I had tried to maintain a balance between respecting Mr. K's role of assessing and diagnosing Earl, and asserting my strong suspicion that Earl had Lewy body dementia.

Mr. K's questions to Earl were probing. He took his time, carefully listening to Earl's responses. He also gave Earl a cognitive exam. He asked Earl to draw a clock, which confused Earl. He could repeat back to Mr. K only one of three words given to him in a list. Earl did not know the day of the week, but he did know the name of the current president. Mr. K then asked Earl how he was feeling. Earl responded that he felt emotionally and mentally "flat," and that his physical balance was off.

Mr. K said he wanted to prescribe two medications he thought would help Earl. One would help him feel less "flat" and one would help with his balance. (I later learned it is best to start only one medication at a time, so if side-effects arise, we can easily determine the medication that caused them.) Mr. K told us he would schedule an appointment for us to see a neurologist, who could confirm if the meds were helpful. I thought this was a clever way for Mr. K to tell us he suspected Lewy body dementia, but that the neurologist would be the one to confirm it.

The way the VA healthcare system works, a patient's primary healthcare provider is responsible for contacting the neurology department to set up an appointment. At the time, I did not know how critical it would be to see a neurologist who was familiar with LBD. I naively believed that all VA neurologists (most of them have a joint appointment, also working at Duke) would be familiar with LBD. I would later learn this was, most certainly, not the case.

Before we left the exam room, Mr. K handed Earl a pamphlet on Lewy body dementia. Earl looked into Mr. K's eyes and said, "Remember what I've told you, no unnecessary treatments."

Mr. K nodded that he understood and respected Earl's wishes.

When we arrived home, Earl read the pamphlet. He said, "We are both going to need support." I took a deep breath and felt grateful. Earl understood what was ahead for the two of us.

We are fortunate that Earl's primary healthcare provider is a physician assistant who is knowledgeable about Lewy body dementia. There are drugs that, in some patients, can stabilize LBD and keep a person from slipping further into the disease. Sometimes the drug works for a few months, on occasion, even longer.

A friend did some investigating of Dr. C, the neurologist we will see in May. She learned Dr. C has been mentored by a doctor at the University of North Carolina Lewy Body Dementia Research Center of Excellence, one of only twenty-six such centers in the U.S. I don't know if Earl's primary healthcare provider specifically requested this neurologist or if we just got lucky. Either way, this is a huge relief!

An LBD diagnosis takes an average of eighteen months and several doctors to pinpoint.[1] LBD is often misdiagnosed due to its shared symptoms with other diseases, such as Alzheimer's and Parkinson's.

Whereas Alzheimer's is associated with memory loss, Lewy body dementia is more about attention dipping in and out, seeing

1. Whiteman, "Lewy Body Dementia," *Medical News Today.*

or hearing things that aren't there, acting out dreams or becoming violent during sleep, and symptoms associated with Parkinson's.[2]

People with LBD either first have symptoms related to cognitive functioning (for example: they can no longer do finances, playing games becomes difficult, they have car accidents because of perception problems, etc.), or their early symptoms look more like Parkinson's (trembling, shuffle-walking, spasms, etc.), with cognitive symptoms appearing later.[3] Earl's early symptoms were mostly related to cognitive functioning.

Because people with LBD tend to fluctuate considerably in mood and lucidity, a person might have a scheduled appointment with a medical person and be having a "good" day, referred to as "showtime." When this happens, the medical professional could miss many signs of LBD.

I'm delighted to report that the mood drug Earl is taking has lifted him out of his listlessness and apathy. He is engaging in more conversations, helping me in the kitchen, and he even vacuumed today.

The turn-around in his mood and level of activity is remarkable. Of course, this won't last long. The average for the drug to be helpful is six months. I'm soaking up every bit of this time I can.

Earl's sense of humor about having Lewy is dear. I'm working hard to help him separate himself from Lewy symptoms, so when something bizarre occurs, he can contribute it to Lewy. Hopefully, as the disease advances, this will help him know it's Lewy and not himself who is "to blame."

Earl's attitude about his diagnosis is, "Well, we all have to die someway." He is not fearful of death. I've spent days and weeks reading and educating myself about the disease. Earl asks me many questions about LBD and he is heartened by my knowledge. He knows he has an advocate by his side.

2. Lewy Body Dementia Association, "Symptoms," *Lbda.org.*
3. Lewy Body Society, "Symptoms," *Lewybody.org.*

We plan to start attending a dementia support group for couples at Duke this month. I keep thinking about the many years we benefited from Marriage Enrichment groups, and hope this experience will also be valuable to us.

LBD is often referred to as "the monster" because of the fluctuations in mood it causes. Caregivers never know "who" is going to show up from day to day, or hour to hour. People with LBD can have auditory and visual hallucinations, and rapid eye movement (REM) sleep problems. Also, the Parkinsonian symptoms will continue to get worse. Although there are stages of LBD, symptoms vary significantly among individuals. It is a roller-coaster ride. We can't ever really know what to expect. I must remain on my toes for whatever symptoms come our way.

Despite all these challenges, I'm not a fan of the word "monster." This way of describing the disease may be accurate, but it does not help me or Earl focus on getting through each day as best we can.

Here are the steps I'm currently taking for self-care:

1. Two daily walks, often accompanied by Earl on one of them.

2. Spend time with a friend once or twice a week.

3. I had intended to participate in an online LBD caregivers support group. I gave it a try, but did not find it helpful, because people in the group seemed to focus on the hard days and shared little about the days of gratitude. It's bad for my mental health to only focus on the challenges and difficulties. It helps me to focus on the positive. I'm grateful the group exists, and I hope it is helpful for others, but it wasn't my cup of tea.

4. An upcoming appointment for Earl and me with an attorney who specializes in elder care, to review our legal documents such as our wills and powers of attorney.

5. An appointment with a social worker at the VA to learn about the benefits Earl is entitled to as the disease progresses.

6. A long-time friend is arriving tonight from upstate New York. She is house-sitting for my daughter and her family while they travel. My friend plans to help me by spending time with Earl, who she knows well, so I can take some respite time and make several appointments for myself.

7. For fun, I joined the Museum of Life and Science, which is within walking distance from our home.

I made a lovely new connection. I received an email from Pat Snyder, who wrote *Treasures in the Darkness: Extending the Early Stage of Lewy Body Dementia, Alzheimer's, and Parkinson's Disease*, a very helpful book.[4] She lives not far from Durham and invited me to meet her for lunch. Her husband of forty-seven years died from LBD last year.

I was delighted Pat reached out. I enjoyed our lunch together. Pat offered me her support and assured me that I was up for the challenge ahead. Her experience with diagnosis—she and her husband saw many medical professionals before a correct diagnosis—was so different from our experience. It doubles my gratitude for Earl's primary healthcare provider, who acknowledged the troubling symptoms, did his research on LBD, and set us up with a neurologist who, fortunately, is knowledgeable about LBD.

Right now, this minute, Earl and I are doing well. I hope you are, too.

Love,
Juanita

---

4. Snyder, *Treasures in the Darkness*.

April 6, 2019

Greetings Dear Ones,

Earl recently sent an email to his 1960's army buddy and wrote, "Despite my diagnosis, Juanita and I are happy." I suppose we are.

The medications Earl began taking in early March have offered us some more time to enjoy one another. He has gone from listless and apathetic to alert and engaged, although often confused. His body tremors are fewer and hallucinations are less frequent.

We have a daily routine, which seldom changes, because Earl does best with consistency. He is dependent on me, and has the expectation I can take care of him and love him. I've told him I'm his second brain, which seems to reassure him.

I'm surprised at the depth of love I'm experiencing for Earl. I suspect many people who become carers of a loved one experience this curious phenomenon. This caregiving role is demanding. Some days, and nights, it sucks everything out of me. But love does endure, even grow. A sense of humor helps, too.

Earl and I hold hands more often. I soothe him when he is agitated in his sleep. I tuck him in when he goes to bed, oh, so early. I watch him closely when we take a walk, in case he trips. I do all of these small things with love and care. I feel no resentment for how our life is now. Instead, despite concern and not knowing what is to come, I feel a powerful love for this man who is so gracefully losing his cognitive functioning and his body. I know our lives will get much harder. This could happen quickly, or slowly over time.

Earl speaks openly to his friends about his diagnosis. He doesn't like to be anywhere but home, so at least twice a week, I arrange for a friend to visit him. When one friend admonished Earl for not making more of an effort to get to a group he has participated in for many years, Earl gave the person a synopsis of what Lewy is like. He told him that his symptoms are like being on a roller coaster, and from minute to minute, hour to hour, he doesn't know how he will feel. I'm proud of how Earl is able to advocate for himself and educate his friends.

Earl's openness and acceptance of what he is experiencing is a gift to both of us. There is no "elephant" we must ignore in our home. We converse often about what is being taken from him. And, he knows I will be okay. He is thankful he has children who love him and can accept what is happening to him with their own grace, compassion, and sorrow. We are fortunate our daughter saw Earl's early symptoms of cognitive decline, and urged us to move next door to her, our son-in-law, and grandson.

Earl has responded to a request from researchers at North Carolina State University (NCSU) to participate in a dementia study, sponsored by the National Health Organization (NHO). As much as Earl dislikes public spaces, he wants to be a part of this study. Isn't it interesting—supervising clinical trials is what he did professionally, and now he will be participating in an NHO study as a participant.

The year-long Museum of Life and Science membership I purchased for myself has been a blessing. When I can, I walk to the museum and head for a bench by the pond, where great blue herons, ducks, geese, and bullfrogs gather. The trees are lush, and there is plenty of shade. Sometimes I take a book along, but often I simply breathe slowly in and out and say, "I am grateful for this life; may I have strength for the journey ahead."

This morning, Earl asked me if it was too much work for me to care for him. He said he only wanted palliative care, and did not want either of us to suffer. He is such a kind, thoughtful soul. I want to be that kind to him, too.

While our son Rich, who lives in Oregon, was visiting, Rich, Jen, and I found a private time to share our concerns with each other, and make a plan for going forward. Because their father has been so clear that he does not want unnecessary treatments and has no fear of death, it was easy for us to agree we would honor his wishes. There will be no interventions to extend Earl's life.

There have been three new wrinkles:

1. Earl asked me to not tell him our plans for the day. In other words, if someone is coming to visit, he doesn't want to know ahead of time.

2. Today's walk was so arduous for Earl that I think it may have been his last.

3. When I reminded Earl about the dementia support group for couples at Duke, he made a face and said, "You can go if you think it would help. But I have no interest in that." I am not surprised that he has decided not to go, but I am very disappointed. I was really looking forward to connecting with couples who are in a similar situation.

Hug someone you care for today and tell them how important they are to you.

May you be well,
Juanita

June 9, 2019

Dear Loved Ones,

Today is our fifty-fourth wedding anniversary, and Earl's seventy-eighth birthday. We had looked forward to going to our Unitarian fellowship together this morning, and then out for lunch. But Lewy intervened.

Earl fell last night, hitting his head on the wall. We can expect many falls. It is one of the hallmarks of Parkinsonism in LBD. Earl's falls scare us both.

Earl is still strong and able to get himself up. When he was upright, sitting on a chair, I checked his eyes for clarity, and his head for any injury. Then Earl found a spot on the sofa in the "kitty-cat" sunlight and said he would rest for a while.

Thinking about the fact this was our anniversary, my thoughts wandered to when we met in college, and the Friday night dances we so enjoyed . . . and the stark contrast between then and where we are now.

Earl says he will rest today. He is sore and unsteady. I'm disappointed to miss church and our anniversary lunch. I mean extremely disappointed! I need to be with people—and somewhere different than inside this house.

I've had to learn to be flexible in my responses, which is not easy for someone who likes to make a plan and stick to it. I don't think I could survive this "every day is different" disease without humor, empathy, and love.

Earl has given up using his iPhone. It is too confusing. I looked into finding him a simpler, "senior-friendly" cellphone with big buttons and limited functions. They do exist, but I thought the odds of Earl using one was low. We have tried a landline phone with a large keypad, with photos of people to speed-dial, but this was also too confusing. I'd like for him to be able to reach people, but someone is with him almost all the time. We need to choose peace over frustration.

My last update mentioned Earl had been accepted into a dementia study at NCSU. He had his first visit with the investigators two weeks ago. Earl spent three hours answering questions and taking written tests. He enjoyed himself immensely. Through the wall, I could hear him laughing at his errors. He doesn't apologize for what he no longer knows. Instead, he will say, "Lewy has come to visit." Bless him, he doesn't seem to be experiencing any shame, only astonishment.

As we left the university, Earl, the Ph.D. biostatistician, said to me, "Can you believe it? They wanted me to add a number, and then subtract a number. Who can do that?"

Every week, we receive a questionnaire from the dementia study for Earl to report how he is doing. It turns out my reading him the questions is a terrific way for us to talk about his feelings, which is an unexpected bonus for us both. In six months, he will return to NCSU for another interview.

There is exciting news out of Georgetown University, where they are going to begin a phase-two trial of a cancer drug that looks promising for people with LBD. At Earl's urging, I wrote to the investigator. It appears Earl meets all the criteria. They would like to include him in their small study of thirty people. It would mean six (six!) visits to Georgetown over a sixteen-week period. Earl suggested we stay with a friend in Fredericksburg and take the train into D.C. for the visits—as if that would be easy! He gave no consideration as to how we would get to Fredericksburg, which is a three- or four-hour drive from where we live.

Fortunately, after further thought, Earl acknowledged it would be too hard to do. I was so relieved. Going to NCSU, which is only forty minutes away, is already very tiring for Earl. I'm grateful he can understand how difficult it would be to travel to D.C. six times in sixteen weeks.

Luckily, if the phase-two trial is successful, there will be multiple locations for LBD patients to participate in phase three. At that juncture, Earl is hopeful he could participate at Duke.

Last week, I attended a caregivers' summit in Durham. The primary reason I went was to participate in a "virtual dementia" tour. I hoped it would increase my understanding of what Earl sometimes experiences. One day, one hour—cognition can fluctuate dramatically.

Here is my account of the "virtual dementia" tour:

I was instructed to put sharp spikes on the soles of my feet, then put on: my shoes, heavy work gloves three sizes too big, dark glasses with no side vision and a narrow vision path straight ahead, and a headset that was constantly muttering—people talking in the distance, or a telephone ringing, a siren—always some kind of annoying sound.

After I put on all the gear, a volunteer took me into a dimly lit room and read me twelve instructions. They stood at my side instead of facing me. They only read the list once. I had to remember what they said and figure out what to do.

First, I had to put on a jacket. The dim light and dark glasses made it very difficult to see. I found a table with clothes on it. After groping around, I found something that felt like it had arms, but I couldn't get it on because of the huge gloves, so I wrapped it around my shoulders. Then I was supposed to set a table for twelve. I found dishes and silverware on a table, but couldn't manipulate the stuff because of the gloves. I laughed with embarrassment at the lousy job I was doing. I thought about how easily someone could feel ashamed and become irritated. All this time, there was rambling chatter in the headset.

After I had set the table in some fashion, I knew there were other things I was supposed to do, but I had no clue what they were.

I stood alone, listened to the chatter, and cursed the darned spikes in my shoes that were killing my feet.

After the "tour" was over, I processed the experience with a dementia specialist. The spikes in the shoes were to simulate body pain, and how people compensate for the pain. The glasses simulated the vision problems people have. The gloves demonstrated how difficult it is to dress oneself due to physical decline. The chatter and noise in the headset demonstrated how troubling sounds can be. The long list of things to do, instructed from the side, demonstrated the importance of standing in front of a person, making eye contact, and giving one instruction at a time.

The experience did me in! I was so sad, and utterly exhausted, but with a new reserve of empathy. I hope I can hold onto the compassion and empathy the "virtual dementia" tour taught me.

In closing, let me return to today: our anniversary and Earl's birthday. Earl has never been a gift-giver, but today he gave me a hug, and asked me if I would like some new jewelry. The question surprised me and brought back what is now a fond memory. On our anniversary decades ago, we went out for breakfast with our friends, June and Doug. Earl pulled a jewelry box out of his pocket and presented me with a very sparkly necklace, one I would never choose for myself. He was so pleased with his gift. I can guarantee it was an effort for him to buy it. It was so out of character.

June, with eyes as big as saucers, giggled when she saw the necklace. She covered her mouth, trying to keep quiet. She knew the necklace was not something I would ever choose for myself. Doug politely complemented Earl on his gift, which caused June to shoot me a knowing look.

I wore the necklace on a few occasions, making a point of thanking Earl for his gift. I knew the purchase had been made with the best of intentions, even though it missed the mark.

Earl rallied today, and we did go out for lunch! He always asks me to order for him and pay. But because it was our anniversary, Earl insisted on ordering our food and paying for our lunch himself. It was a small thing, but in our new world, a sweet, sweet gesture. Much better than a sparkly piece of jewelry.

Sending love and light your way,
Juanita

August 2, 2019

Greetings Friends and Family,

From a nurse who visited our home, we learned of a VA provision that funds bathroom improvements. I contacted Earl's primary healthcare provider to ask for a referral, which took us to the VA's Occupational Therapy Clinic. Earl and I spent an hour with a fantastic occupational therapist who understands LBD well. She was such a help to Earl; she was knowledgeable and empathetic.

Earl cried. He told her, "I used to be sharp as a tack, now I fumble for words."

I took with me pictures of our bathtub and pointed out the dangers the tub and shower present for Earl, especially stepping in and out. The occupational therapist submitted a request for us to receive financial assistance to take out the tub and put in a walk-in shower. I'm learning the importance of advocating—with documentation!

There have been a few pretty big bumps in the road since my last update.

I love my morning walks. But I returned home one morning from my walk to find Earl in a panic. He had had an auditory hallucination that I was yelling for help. He imagined I had fallen and had been run over by a car.

Even after I calmed him down, he continued to insist that I immediately purchase pepper spray, and always carry it in my hand (not just in a pocket) when I walk in our neighborhood. He would not relent. Finally, I said I would. Telling him I didn't need it only escalated his agitation. This gave me a frightening glimpse of how difficult it might become for me to continue going on my much-needed, sanity-saving walks.

Earl has had some rough nights recently, when auditory and/or visual hallucinations interfere with his (our) sleep. One night, at 3 AM, we stood together at a window while Earl told me what he was hearing and seeing for a very l-o-n-g time.

I have a mantra for these nights: "This is Lewy visiting us, all will be well." This mantra, and mindful breathing, are helpful.

So, the two of us continue to figure things out. I'm getting better at listening to Earl tell me what he wants, and what he doesn't want, and how he wants to contribute. I have realized, in wanting to protect him and keep him safe, I was taking away some of his autonomy. I'm doing better at recognizing when I do that.

We have spent the hot North Carolina summer immersed in British mysteries on TV. From *Endeavor* to *Morse* to *Lewis*, we have rewatched them all. Although sometimes it feels like a task to rewatch these mysteries (I remember most of the episodes, Earl does not), it provides us with entertainment on hot summer afternoons. After watching all of the above series, we restarted the first episode of *Foyle's War* and devoured all of them, too.

It was a pleasure to see Earl enjoy the stories. When we finished an episode, we talked about what we had watched. In the case of *Foyle's War*, Earl enhanced each episode with his own knowledge, having studied the history of World War II.

Our dear friends Dale and Sandy, from our Fredericksburg years, traveled from their home in Ohio in order to spend just two hours with us (Earl's limit for socializing), and then turned around to head home. My friend June, from New York, drove ten hours to spend time with Earl so I could attend important meetings and get my teeth cleaned. Brenda, a friend from Fredericksburg, who has relatives in NC, came out of her way to have lunch with me and bring me delicious chocolates. And both of Earl's nieces, Susan and Linda, and their husbands, have made an effort to travel great distances to spend time with us.

I must carefully plan these visits. Earl prefers I not tell him about visitors ahead of time, but that doesn't work when guests are traveling from afar.

We can no longer accommodate out-of-town guests overnight in our home, something I always used to enjoy. It's just too much for Earl.

For the most part, Earl does enjoy seeing special friends and family. However, there have been two occasions when I have had to cancel a visit from someone coming from out of town. The cancellations were because Earl was agitated, knowing his routine would need to change that day. It distresses me when I have to advise a friend, who has traveled from elsewhere, that it is not a good day for a visit.

People are kind and generous with their time. He is always happy to have Jen come over—that doesn't seem to tire him. Earl does have a limit as to how long he enjoys having other visitors, but he has agreed to let me arrange for him to have company so I can continue to attend my book group. Friend visits are very helpful for me, too. Some friends have stepped up to have meaningful conversations with Earl, including a sixteen-year-old grandchild of a friend, who wanted to ask Earl about his spiritual beliefs.

It is heartwarming and touching to have people respond when I put out a call for help. It's easy for me to recognize that I can't, by myself, provide Earl with the stimulation and richness of conversation he deserves and thrives on. We are blessed with good friends, some old, some new. Interestingly, it is some of the new friends who are most eager to spend time with Earl. Sometimes they tell him something about their lives they may not share with many people. One time, one of the new friends confided in Earl that he was estranged from a family member. When the visitor left, Earl told me what the person had told him.

Earl said, "He probably didn't think I'd remember what he said." We both smiled in acknowledgment.

It means a great deal to me that we can continue to host people in our home. Conversations sometimes take on an urgency, a vulnerability, that is so genuine and real. Our home is being stored up with stories, laughter, and tears. There will come a time when Earl can no longer have visitors, or even converse. I hope the memories of what we are experiencing now will help sustain us both.

Be well, y'all. Give someone you care about a hug today,
Juanita

October 8, 2019

Dear Friends and Family,

Recently, two of Earl's friends visited. Their conversation with Earl helped me understand how mistaken some people are concerning what it means to have LBD. They were amazed that Earl engaged with them in conversation. He laughed with them and recalled past experiences they all had together. I felt I had had a glimpse of how misunderstood dementia with Lewy is, with the surprised responses from the two visitors.

When someone asks me what it is like to live with someone with dementia, the assumption is often that it is only sorrow and decline. But that is misinformed. Alongside the losses are tenderness, sweet rituals, and moments of deep connection.

Earl's initial visit to see a new dentist, one who has a practice closer to where we live, illustrates the way that many people tend to treat people who have dementia: condescending to them as if they were children. I had made sure the dentist and hygienist were comfortable treating someone with LBD before I made an appointment for Earl; when we arrived at the office for the first time, they knew Earl's diagnosis.

The dental hygienist who ushered Earl from the waiting room seemed to infantilize him. She called Earl "baby doll" several times. Earl finally said to her, "I would prefer you call me Dr. Johnson," at which point the hygienist giggled. I quietly repeated that Earl would like to be called Dr. Johnson. The hygienist looked at me and said, "For real?"

It was nice to see Earl calmly asserting himself, to maintain his dignity. The hygienist apologized, saying she was raised in the south and calls everyone "baby doll," but ever since that encounter, Earl is referred to as Dr. Johnson at the dentist's office.

We have had two other recent encounters with medical professionals. The first was a second appointment with the occupational therapist. Once again, she was incredibly helpful to Earl, listening carefully and sharing useful tips on how he could make his daily life easier. She told Earl he was brave for acknowledging his disease. She was surprised by his comfort discussing Lewy. She asked us to please inform her of ways we navigate LBD together; she felt we could offer help to others with the disease. Then she told Earl he was "forty percent ahead of the game," which we took to mean that the way he is accepting what he has makes things easier for him (and certainly for his family, as well).

When we saw the neurologist, he again told Earl that he was impressed with Earl's "pleasant affect." He said it was unusual for him to see someone with LBD who was accepting the diagnosis with "humor and grace." The neurologist never hurries us, so I turned to face Earl, took his hands in mine, and asked him to repeat what the doctor had said to him about his pleasant affect and his humor and grace. I wanted to be sure the words sunk in.

The doctor said it was impressive how Earl and I can talk about the disease together, pay attention to new symptoms, and be proactive. Words of encouragement are so important for patients and caregivers to hear.

Earl believes his fifteen years practicing the principles of *A Course in Miracles* has impacted his present response to LBD.[1] I wish you could all witness first-hand how kind and thoughtful he often is to me. He tells me it takes effort: he has to work really hard to respond in kind ways, and some days it is nearly impossible. But he tries.

---

1. Schucman, *A Course in Miracles*.

Earl's most challenging times, at least for right now, come during the night. As is common with Lewy, there is a lot of movement of the body during REM sleep, and often terrifying dreams that can be acted out. There have been a couple of incidents where I have been frightened when Earl's strong arms and body have caused me to be in some danger. He pushed me out of bed one night. Another time, Earl pulled my hair, trying to hold on to me. With each of these episodes, my shouting, "Stop!" immediately brought him awake, with an instant apology.

One night, while in REM sleep, he put a pillow over my face. It was terrifying. I have moved to sleeping in a different bed in order to be safe.

However, every night around 4 AM, when I know the REM sleep has passed, I slip into bed with Earl. I snuggle up close to him, breathe deeply, and have the best sleep of my night.

It is a good discipline to practice living in the moment. Lewy is so unique to each person, it is impossible to predict day to day, let alone the future. As a planner, it is often very hard for me to stick to just "what is." A friend pointed out that I like teaching others about the benefits of presence, and living in the moment, and maybe now I can experience that firsthand. Let me assure you, it takes discipline to accept, and be present, to just embrace the day you have in front of you.

I continue to learn what it means to be a care partner. One thing is for sure, no matter where I am, I'm thinking about Earl. It's like a little nugget in the back of the head that just never goes away. I've also learned it is exhausting to care so much and always be attuned to what is happening with Earl. And friends, we are only in the early days of this disease.

But here's the thing. I think this diagnosis has brought out the very best in both of us. It's surprising the growth and changes I'm experiencing. I am enjoying Earl in ways I've never appreciated before. We are good buddies on this last ride, weaving our hearts together. I don't know that I can articulate how amazing this is to me.

Tell a loved one you care,
Juanita

October 11, 2019

One of the medications Earl was on, when the doctor increased the dosage, caused Earl to become aggressive in wanting to have sex.

Frankly, this aggression was disturbing.

I could show him affection with hand holding and a good-night kiss—but I had my limits.

I did not wait until the neurologist gave permission to reduce the dosage.

No, I immediately reduced the dose to what it had been before. Then I contacted the doctor and told him what I had done.

This is not the only time I took the initiative to reduce a dose or even stop a medication when Earl had an adverse reaction. Another medication made him very dizzy and thus more likely to fall. I stopped that one immediately. The neurologist has been quite surprised at the adverse reactions Earl has had to some of the medicines. He told me that care partners often have a better understanding of how effective a medication is because they are with the patient on a daily basis. I felt respected—and relieved—that the neurologist responded well to my being proactive.

December 2, 2019

Dear Friends and Family,

It has been almost a year since Earl was officially diagnosed with LBD, although in retrospect, he had symptoms as early as three years prior to the diagnosis.

During this past year, I've shifted into the role of full-time care partner. It took me a while to acknowledge that my life, and our lives, had changed. At first, I tried to make Earl better by correcting him, and reminding him he knew how to do whatever was troubling him. What an utter waste of time that was, and disrespectful of Earl.

I was such a mess at first that our daughter thought she would need to care for both her mom and her dad. I was in denial, or I was angry, or I was grieving—sometimes all at once.

Care-partnering is a burden, and it is lonesome. My glass can be half empty or half full. It's my choice. Eleanor Roosevelt wrote, "One's philosophy is not best expressed in words, it is expressed in the choices one makes . . . . And the choices we make are ultimately our own responsibility."[1] I have been blessed with a resilient and positive outlook. I never considered how helpful these characteristics could be as a care partner. I'm researching and reading about the disease and how others have walked this path. I continue to learn how I can best assist Earl.

I'm responsible for everything in our lives. A social worker who recently visited us put it this way. She said, "In a relationship, there is give and take. Sometimes one of you gives 70%, the other

1. Roosevelt, *You Learn by Living*, unpaginated foreword.

30%. Other times this shifts. But now you are responsible for 100% of the relationship." She also told me that my positive attitude, my smile, and my respect for Earl help both of us now and will continue to as Earl declines. Boy, did I soak up those affirming words.

"Lewy" shows up when a "trigger" has been pushed. It might be loud noises from outside or listening to a news update. It could be an elastic band at Earl's waist, or that his comfy socks are not comfy. Or the trigger might be a headache or an infection. My job is to locate the trigger as quickly as possible, do what I can to mitigate it, and try to soothe with distraction: music, a hug, ice cream, or a nap.

Occasionally the trigger is obvious. Other times, it's only in retrospect that I can figure out what caused Lewy to show up.

Yes, it's exhausting, sometimes scary, sometimes sad.

One of my early hard days was a day Earl was listening to a news broadcast on National Public Radio. Afterwards, he confronted me. He said with an angry voice, "I'm going to get a car for myself if you don't let me drive yours." He was belligerent, standing close and leering. His voice petrified me. Rationally, I realized the news had triggered the outburst. But I still felt defenseless and very, very frightened. I stammered something about finding someone who could help him look for a car—hoping and praying this notion would pass. It did pass. But I was really scared: of his voice, his stance, his eyes.

When I was a little girl, an only child, I had an imaginary companion named Gerda. When I felt confused, lonesome, or sad, she was by my side. At some point in growing into middle childhood, I bade goodbye to Gerda. I hoped she would find another child to befriend.

Recently, I was sharing with my friend Rae what happens in my body when Lewy shows up. Lewy has a distinct voice: an accusing, harsh voice. I do not have skin as tough as a rhino! That voice causes me to break out into a sweat and my tummy begins to do cartwheels. As I described what this was like for me, Rae said, "That sounds like fear." Bingo! Then the question was, what can I do to care for myself when I am afraid? How can I feel safe? It made me think of my imaginary friend Gerda, and the comfort and nurturing she brought me as a child. I'm pleased to tell you Gerda has returned to accompany me through these troubling times. Her return has offered me much comfort, and she makes me smile. Even an imaginary friend can offer support.

Additionally, I have been learning how to shift attention to other parts of my body, away from the distressed parts, when I'm in a difficult or scary situation. Concentrating on my breathing (breathe in for a count of five, breathe out for a count of five) helps. Of course, if I felt I was in real physical danger, I would leave the house, and call someone to join me before going back inside.

For the most part, our days go smoothly. Good days are comfortable, we are content. Earl's acceptance of his disease makes such a difference in the ease of our days. Last Sunday afternoon, out of the blue, Earl told me how much my "Let's make the most of this day" attitude helped him on hard days. This disease shrinks a person's capacity to show kindness for their care partner. It was remarkable he could say such a thing to me.

We have never had an easy marriage. There have been gentle years and difficult ones, but through it all, we shared a commitment to keep growing—spiritually, emotionally, and in how we loved each other. We didn't always get it right, but we kept trying to understand one another more fully. Now, in these later years, we lean on what love and time have taught us.

Adversity has driven me deeper. It has made me kinder. There is a tenderness I feel for Earl that fills me with such love.

Our worlds have shrunk. Earl no longer wants to go anywhere, except to get his hair cut once a month. He really enjoys the time with his hairdresser, who just happens to be young and attractive. Afterwards, we go to our favorite diner for a late breakfast. Haircut days are special days.

Earl had been continuing to mostly enjoy visits from friends—until recently, when he asked for a "sabbatical" from having visitors. He says he knows it's good to be social, but maybe that is more for people with Alzheimer's than Lewy. He may have a point. He said he is sorry I don't have more opportunities for fun.

Nothing is spontaneous. I'm determined to continue to connect with my friends and hold on to myself. But it takes effort to make this happen.

I have been reading Pauline Boss' book, *Ambiguous Loss*.[2] She writes about living with someone you love who is still alive—but lost to us nevertheless. Boss emphasizes the need to build resilience in order to live with uncertainty, which seems sage advice.

I've thought a great deal about how Earl and I were able to meet his diagnosis head on, and move forward as a team. I believe our resilient attitudes have made a significant difference. For us, resilience means being honest about what is happening—there has been no denial. We have tried to stay calm. I research and study the illness and share what I learn with Earl. Together, we have learned to be flexible when our daily lives need to change. I practice patience, and I try to acknowledge both what I can do and where my limits are. Strengthening my resilience is one of the factors that allows me to keep showing up, even on the hardest days.

Earl is falling more frequently. Falling can happen when he doesn't pick his feet up and trips, or if he bends over and tries to stand up too quickly, or from getting dizzy. We have eliminated rugs or sealed them to the wood floor with rug tape. And yet, he still finds ways to fall. So far, he has managed to get himself up. He has not been injured. But you can imagine my reluctance in leaving him alone.

What am I going to do when Earl can no longer get up from a fall by himself? He weighs more than me. I know I would hurt myself trying to lift him. I'm investigating devices that I may need to have on hand.

The VA is providing us with small cameras to use in our home, which will connect to my phone. If I'm not home, I'll be able to check the cameras. My daughter, next door, will also be

2. Boss, *Ambiguous Loss: Learning to Live with Unresolved Grief.*

able to monitor them. The VA has also supplied us with a fall/panic button. Somehow this does not offer me much reassurance that he will be okay when I am not home. Perhaps I'll find these technologies more helpful than I think?

Instead of cameras or alarms, I'd much rather know someone is with Earl when I'm not. Fortunately, our daughter is usually able to come over when I need respite time. It gives me peace of mind, because both Earl and I trust that Jen will keep him safe.

Earl always enjoys his daughter when she visits. But Jen tells me that every time they are together, after an hour or so, her dad walks to the front door and stands at the full-window storm door, watching and waiting for me to come home. No matter what Jen says, or how much she reassures him that I will be back soon, he stands at the door, waiting.

We are blessed to have children and a son-in-law who have stepped up in their own unique ways to be supportive and helpful.

I really felt the loss of family rituals at Halloween. We have always carved pumpkins with Jen, Noah, and Sam. We didn't join them this year because knives and carving would be dangerous. Earl has always insisted we buy full-sized candy bars for trick-or-treaters. He would sit on our front porch to greet the children. This year, to keep our house calm and predictable for Earl, I kept our porch light off, no full-sized candy bars given out. Another loss.

Thanksgiving, Earl and I stayed in our home and had a small turkey dinner, just the two of us. Our family joined us for dessert. It was surprisingly okay. Christmas, who knows? All familiar rituals are up in the air. What matters most is keeping life peaceful, with as few disruptions to Earl's routine as possible.

Our grandson, who enjoys family rituals as much as I do, is feeling our absence and the changes. Fortunately, he and I continue to bake together in our kitchen. Really, I just chat with him while he bakes; he has become an excellent baker. One holds on to the rituals that one can.

My daughter lovingly asked me what my personal expectations are for the holidays. Sure, there is a feeling of loss, and to some degree, disconnection from our family. But for now, it's about Earl's comfort, nothing trumps that. I can journal about my feelings or talk with a friend. But truthfully, unless you've been through it, no one can really understand how isolating caregiving can be.

One of my frequent reminders to my students was that the ability to be flexible in one's expectations, especially as one ages, is a key factor in enjoying life. I keep reminding myself of that, and it helps. Bottom line: under the circumstances, we are doing quite well. Earl and I find comfort in the ordinary.

Yesterday, I told Earl breakfast was ready and I would help him get up and get dressed. He asked me to stand in front of him when talking to him. I was surprised he asked me to stand in front of him. I remembered I'm supposed to do that with someone with dementia, but the fact he recognized it would be helpful was interesting.

When I was in position, Earl said, "The snowstorm has stopped in my bedroom, and the horse is back in his stall, so I guess I can get up." He chuckled—and I knew from the twinkle in his eyes that he recognized this had been a dream, not a hallucination. We both joyfully laughed. A glorious sacred moment!

Let me wrap up these musings with a favorite quote from Thich Nhat Hahn: "Cherish this very moment. Let go of the streams of distress and embrace life fully in your arms."[3]

Love,
Juanita

P.S. Fun fact: I will be seventy-five years young on December tenth. I will, with pleasure, accept cards, emails, texts, dark chocolate, and good wishes. Please, no phone calls. We have a small home and calls can be disruptive.

---

3. Thich Nhat Hanh, *Call Me by my True Names*, 226.

The Middle Time: January 2020–January 2021

Daily Rhythms of Care

The start of each morning is a delicate time. I'm still up early—showered and dressed by 7:30, moving quietly through the house. Earl wakes around 8:00. It takes him a few minutes to be fully awake.

I try to offer Earl a cheerful greeting to orient him to the day: "Good morning, Sunshine. It's a chilly winter day. We are in our home in North Carolina, next door to Jen-Pooh, Noah, Sam, and their dog, Pepper. Rich is asleep in his home in Oregon, where it is still nighttime. Everyone is safe and comfortable." Earl takes this all in.

He walks to the bathroom on his own and insists on washing his face and brushing his teeth. These are small victories I don't take for granted.

Dressing has become slower and more difficult for Earl. I lay out soft clothes that slip on easily—pants with elastic waistbands that don't itch or pinch. I bless the day I found an orange clothing marker pen—it became a tiny miracle, enabling me to mark the inside back of his shirts and pants with an orange mark. I bought him socks that have "R" and "L" stitched in. His shoes close with Velcro. I encourage him to do what he can, but I'm always nearby.

Around 9:00 AM, we sit down to a simple breakfast. Earl prefers oatmeal and an orange, sliced into finger-sized pieces. After we eat, he no longer wants to do things alone. "Stay," he says, and so I stay. We listen to music or an audiobook—always together. He still tries to use the iPad, but more often than not, it frustrates him. For a brief, shining window, he was able to read again. I celebrated that moment like a holiday. It didn't last, but it mattered.

Lunch comes at noon. I now serve his lunch, a sandwich and fruit he can pick up with his fingers, on a red plastic plate. I've read that the color red helps people with dementia see their food more clearly. The plates have a lip around the edge, so nothing spills. I've found silverware designed for tremors and a sippy cup with a lid. Small adjustments. Quiet dignity.

Afternoons are a toss-up. Earl sometimes welcomes visitors, sometimes not. I try to sense his energy before confirming anything. Our daughter, who works from home, often visits after lunch.

However, in late March, Covid-19 arrives. All visiting stops.

After Covid-19, it is always just the two of us in our home. Jen's husband works in primary care, and we just can't risk Earl or I being exposed to the virus. We are all tremendously eager for a vaccine.

At 2:00 PM, it's time for our daily nap. My sock feet go in his lap, at his request. My feet are his "fidget board" of sorts. He rubs them until he falls asleep. I stay still, reading or dozing, not wanting to disturb him.

By 3:30 PM, we sit on the front porch if the weather allows. It is our one opportunity to see our neighbors—from a distance. Sometimes Jen, Noah, Sam, or our next-door neighbor, Amy, sit in the front yard for a social-distance visit. If we need to stay inside, we listen to music or an audiobook. I encourage Earl to take a 4:00 PM shower, his preferred time, but often, it doesn't happen. If he doesn't have a shower, he watches TV while I prepare supper for 5:30.

Earl will sometimes randomly decide to shower at a different time of the day. Anytime he wants to shower is a win. I always accommodate his preference.

If Lewy gives him a break, we chat. By 6:30 PM, we watch another TV program. We hold hands, sitting on the couch together.

I've heard alarming stories about "sundowning," which is when people with dementia can become agitated and have a terribly hard time settling down in the late afternoon or evening. I am incredibly thankful that Earl does not experience "sundowning." Just a gradual descent into nighttime. Tooth brushing in the evenings has become increasingly rare, but is still self-managed.

By 8:00 PM, he is in pajamas, in bed. At 8:15 PM, I read a short story and offer a brief meditation. Then I turn on the white-noise machine, kiss him goodnight on his cheek, tell him, "I'll see you in the morning light," and quietly leave.

Phone calls and Zoom meetings confuse him. Earl becomes anxious if he hears me talking to someone he can't see. Our one-story home is quite small; there is little privacy. I've stopped trying to have phone or Zoom conversations. Both of our worlds are shrinking. But his sense of comfort matters most. Each day brings small losses and small graces. And I meet them with a heart that is stretched to straining, but not broken.

February 6, 2020

Dear Friends,

An intuitive friend recently emailed me, asking if an update wasn't overdue. She wondered if that meant caregiving had gotten more challenging. Yes, it has!

Sometimes days are really hard—those are the times when I'm grateful for soil to put my hands in, and plants and flowers to watch grow inside our home. A stillness finds its way into my scattered brain, which helps me focus on my breathing, which helps me feel more centered. We've never had so many indoor plants as we do now! They offer me delight and comfort.

The Lewy roller coaster is taking more dramatic dips and turns. For the most part, Earl's auditory hallucinations have receded, except for the occasional people interrupting non-existent phone calls, or babies crying. But there are many visual hallucinations, such as spiders on the bedroom ceiling, ants on the wall, bugs in the bathroom, or infants crawling on our lawn and porch. A couple days ago, I was dusting imaginary spiders off the bedroom ceiling with the ceiling fan duster. Another day, I assured Earl I had gathered up the babies he thought were on our front porch, and I had gently seen to it that they all got home safely. Sometimes I do feel creative as I search for ways to reassure, and take care of, what is troubling him when Lewy is present.

However, these visual hallucinations, and the less-frequent auditory hallucinations, exhaust both of us. I am fortunate Earl does not wander out of the house, as some with Lewy do. It's the vigilance, though, that wears on me. What will happen next? Being constantly on alert for symptoms, and how I respond to them—always with respect—takes its toll.

When people marry, or partner, there is often this unconscious idea they can change the other person. That notion has been on my mind a lot lately, as I know for certain Earl can't change. His abstract thinking has faded. It takes executive skills to make judgments, to change, and to be flexible. For people with LBD, it is the executive skills that are most affected, rather than memory. I must learn to adapt daily, according to what situation is presenting itself. I don't see how one could offer care to someone with Lewy without daily flexibility to change. Yes, it is exhausting!

My dentist recently told me I looked "depleted." I figured if my dentist thought that, I must be a wreck. Apparently, my daughter thought so, too: she has offered to stay with her dad more often, so I can have additional respite time. Our son is coming for a long weekend later this month. Helping their mom, spending time with their dad—I'm grateful for their care of us.

Earl has many good days. He enjoys watching comedies on TV, doing simple word games on his iPad, and reading his daily meditations when he can. He continues to mostly enjoy visits from friends; he always enjoys visits from his family. When our fifteen-year-old grandson pops in, Earl is especially animated. But I see him slowly slipping away. Sometimes I find myself feeling lonesome for what was, but I feel resolved to go with what is, and make the best of it. We are a team and will support one another as best we can on this path. Even as the Lewy road gets harder, there are still small gems that appear.

I'll end this update by sharing a very active Lewy night with you (fortunately these rarely happen) . . . and a gem.

2:00 AM: "Hon, why is the TV on?"

3:00 AM: "Oh no! There is a leak in the bathroom."

4:00 AM: "Juanita, there is someone at the door."

5:30 AM: "Juanita! There is a large cat in the living room and it is making a mess."

7:00 AM: "Honey, there are bugs in the bathroom."

7:10 AM: We crawl wearily into bed together, both exhausted by all the Lewy activity. I say to Earl, "I love you," and he replies, "I'm grateful." We fall into restful sleep.

All relationships have gems. What are the ones you hold dear?

Love,
Juanita

February 20, 2020

Dear Friends and Family,

Many of you have reached out to express your concern after my last update. Some of you who have dealt with dementia suggested a change in medications, or dosage, might be helpful. I want to assure you that I work closely with our neurologist, who is very responsive.

The reason for this quick update is to share with you that Earl is able to read books again. For several months, his brain hasn't allowed him to concentrate on a narrative for any length of time. For the past several days, he has once again been able to enjoy his very favorite pastime. It fills us both with sunshine and joy!

This is the mysterious path of Lewy. One week, I see a person who is clearly declining. The next, I see a person who is engaged in conversations and reading books! It is why life with Lewy is called "riding the roller coaster." There is no pattern from one day to the next, or even from one person to another, as to how the disease progresses.

On another positive note, Earl has completed the six-month clinical study at NCSU. The study examined cognition, aging, and social awareness. Earl's participation was a tough go, as it meant spending three hours at a time at the bustling university, being interviewed and tested. As a person who supervised clinical trials during his professional life, Earl was eager to participate. We are proud and grateful he could do so.

Living one day at a time,
Juanita

April 16, 2020—amid a pandemic

Dear Friends and Family,

Our son Rich was here in February. It was perfect timing, as he was able to gather supplies for us and return to Oregon before traveling became a worry due to Covid-19.

Jen and I took advantage of Rich being here: while he stayed with Earl, Jen and I visited memory-care homes. People with LBD eventually need twenty-four-hour care. Whether to provide that care at home or at a memory-care facility can be a wrenching decision for a family. If a care facility is necessary, people with LBD seem to do best in very small memory-care settings of seven to ten people. Fortunately, North Carolina has such licensed facilities. Not all states do. Jen and I visited three. From the outside, each of the facilities looked like large houses in beautiful, tree-lined neighborhoods. Inside, we saw comfortable bedrooms with large windows, community rooms filled with light, a kitchen in the center of the home, no clutter, soft music playing, laughter, and hugs. All had walking paths outdoors.

We both thought touring such places would make us very sad. We were surprised when our response instead was hope—and relief. We felt reassured by knowing that such well-staffed, beautiful places are nearby.

I conferred with Earl's niece Susan, who administered nursing homes for years, as to how to talk with Earl about the research Jen and I had done. How would Earl respond to us investigating memory-care homes? We were worried.

Susan told us the family member who lives furthest away should take the lead in discussing difficult topics with someone with dementia. She said, that way, if the person becomes angry, they are not angry with their caregiver or family who live nearby. She suggested Jen, Rich, and I talk with Earl together, with Rich taking the initiative. After talking with Rich about this, he chose to talk with his dad alone. After doing so, Rich reported his dad was aware that, medically, it may someday be impossible for me to keep him home. Earl told Rich he hoped I would find a companion after he died, and that we have long-term care insurance in case I can't take care of him at home.

Earl's response was such a relief! After Rich had this conversation with his dad, I've been able to show Earl pictures of the places Jen and I visited. I've asked him if he would like to ride by or tour any of the homes. He says he trusts my judgment. (I realize a facility must have an opening if we need it—that's the tricky part.) To be perfectly candid, the touring, and Earl's responses, have eased my weariness, at least for now. I see a way forward, if needed, and I trust the process.

There may be difficult conversations your family needs to have. Perhaps regarding last wishes or end-of-life care. Do it now. It will give you all peace of mind.

A year ago, I wrote in my journal how difficult it was not to have time alone in my home. Earl didn't want to go anywhere, not even to visit his family next door. I had no alone time. After we both retired, I always welcomed the times Earl went square-dancing, or to a class at OLLI (water-color painting, and history, were his favorites). It felt necessary and rejuvenating to be home alone, to have uninterrupted time to myself.

I've been thinking about the need I had to be in the house alone, and how that need has waned. It has now been since October of 2018 that I was home by myself. I no longer even think about it. An example of how we can adapt, if we are challenged to do so. We can change our perspective. And hey, it only took me more than a year!

These are extraordinary times. Your sheltering in place probably feels much more restrictive than it does to us; we are used to it. It is our way of life. Astronaut Scott Kelly recently wrote a piece for *The New York Times* explaining how important a routine can be at a time like this.[1] He had a daily routine in space and now has one at home. Like Astronaut Kelly, there are habits I've established that help me, help us, keep harmony in a small space. Here are my suggestions, inspired by Kelly's own list:

- Take deep, intentional breaths. Earl and I especially enjoy sharing a deep-breathing ritual at the end of the day.

- Go outside. Take a walk if you can. We love sitting on the front porch.

- Consider your intake of news. We no longer listen to the news on the radio or watch it on TV. To keep up with current events, I read the news for a short period of time—and then move on.

- Eat something just for pleasure. For us, this is an Oreo cookie or two.

- Listen to music. Sometimes we dance in our kitchen.

- Read out loud to each other. I read to Earl every evening.

- Keep a journal—write or draw your thoughts, feelings, and reflections.

- Make it a point to hold hands.

- Express appreciation and love. Try to find a different person to do this to, every day.

- At the end of the day, share gratitude. When I tuck Earl in at night, I always express my gratitude for him, wish him a peaceful night, and tell him I will see him in the morning light.

---

1. Kelly, "I Spent a Year in Space and Have Tips on Isolation," *The New York Times*.

"Acknowledging the preciousness of each day is a good way to live, a good way to reconnect to our basic joy."
—Pema Chodron[2]

Peace and love are flowing your way,
Juanita

P.S. Our nighttime reading is currently *Being Home*, a book of meditations by Gunila Norris.[3]

---

2. Chodron, *The Wisdom of No Escape*, 33.

3. Norris, *Being Home: Discovering the Spiritual in the Everyday.*

May 8, 2020

Dear Family and Friends,

Earl will celebrate his birthday on June ninth. We both very much enjoy receiving cards in the mail. If you are inclined, I know he would love hearing from you. He no longer uses his phone, text, or email.

We speak of many of you on a regular basis. When we reminisce about family gatherings, neighbors past and present, work colleagues, friends, spiritual family, or army buddies, your names pop up. We are grateful for all the ways you have enriched our lives. I've heard a lot of new stories from Earl's life as I gather his oral history, when Lewy takes a hike.

Earl has benefited from the stay-at-home order. I'm with him twenty-four hours a day, and he prefers that. Our routine is basically the same every day. I've been so impressed and appreciative of his flexibility about what we eat. Like many of you, we are ordering our groceries online and often don't get what we want. Earl just goes with the flow.

His sense of humor about "crazy Lewy" has not wavered, even though he is growing more confused, and directions are really hard for him to follow. His walking is unstable, and his eyesight is diminishing.

Fortunately, we continue to be able to have meaningful conversations together. We also enjoy detective shows and documentaries on TV. He had been enjoying reading again, but that is now confusing him. I can see so many ways creative entrepreneurs could design very simple things for people with dementia to use.

His favorite pastime is birdwatching. We have feeders near both our front and back porches. He knows the names of birds and is enchanted watching them. Earl also delights in sitting on our front porch and waving to people walking by. He calls this, "Minding the neighbors' business."

Jen, Sam, and Noah visit with us from a distance outdoors. Sam is expanding his passion for vegetable gardening into our front yard, as we have more sun than their yard. We see him often from our porch, and love to talk with him and watch him maintain his gardens.

We will soon have chickens in our backyard. Noah and Jen have been building a chicken coop for their baby chicks—who are no longer babies. The coop will be in our fenced-in backyard to keep the chickens safely away from their dog. Earl delights in the progression of the project, and we look forward to fresh eggs.

Rich was not able to visit us this month. We are sad not knowing when it may be safe for him to travel here again. For now, we FaceTime and are grateful we can do that. I'm sure many of you are wondering when it will be safe to see your loved ones, as well.

I'm doing okay, despite feeling isolated and really missing my friends.

Phone calls and Zoom continue to confuse Earl. I'm limited in the ways I can connect with others. Text and email are best.

Years ago, I read *Opening Up by Writing It Down* by James Pennebaker and Joshua Smyth.[1] In it, they talk about the therapeutic benefits of expressive writing (journaling); their research demonstrated that regularly writing about traumatic or stressful experiences can improve mental and physical health. Journaling has been incredibly helpful to me over the years. I have used Pennebaker and Smyth's techniques to journal about every emotion imaginable. Right now, writing provides a safe outlet to process and release difficult feelings that arise in me during the day. The

1. Pennbaker and Smyth, *Opening Up by Writing It Down*.

writing helps me gain a different perspective, and it helps relieve some of the stress of caregiving. I can write down distressing thoughts and leave them on the page. I sleep much better after journaling.

I generally have a couple of hours to myself in the evening, and an hour in the morning, which I savor. Knowing I can write in my journal at the end of the day gives me the solace I need to weather whatever the day brings.

On another note, I want to offer a big thank you to those of you locals who occasionally run errands for us. We are so appreciative of your care.

A shout out to the sneaky souls who anonymously leave bouquets of flowers on our front porch. My heart bursts open with flowers in our home. Your thoughtfulness brings me unbounded joy.

In closing, Earl looked at me the other night and said, "You are a really good friend to me."

I replied, "You are my good friend, too, and you make me smile."

And so our journey continues. Thanks for coming along with us.

Warmly,
Juanita

P.S. For those of you who have asked how you could be helpful to us during continuing Covid isolation, here are some suggestions, using online gift cards: Postmates (a food delivery service for local restaurants). Amazon (for bird-feeding supplies and occasional e-books. I utilize our library for e-books, but wait times are sometimes long). The Regulator Bookshop (my favorite local independent bookstore). Subscription to a gardening or journaling magazine. Thank you!

July 16, 2020

Dear Friends and Family,

Thousands of people are caregivers every single day. Many quit or lose their jobs in order to care for a loved one. The quarantine has left others unable to give care or even visit a loved one who is miles away or in a care facility. Will we give caregiving more importance at a national level once the pandemic passes? Some believe we will. Let us hope so.

There is a saying among caregivers that, until you are a caregiver (or care partner), you have no concept of what it is like. "No one gets it." Caregivers often feel adrift and alone.

Writing about my personal experiences feels like a calling. Your reading of my updates offers me support. Please indulge me as I try to put into words what caregiving for someone with LBD is like—for me.

The book *Ten Thousand Joys and Ten Thousand Sorrows* by Olivia Hoblitzelle[1] is my constant companion on this part of the journey. Written from a Buddhist perspective, by a care partner whose spouse had dementia, I find great solace in it. You will find a couple quotes from the book below.

Offering full-time care for Earl, I often need to step back from time to time, to recognize how much energy it takes. Hoblitzelle writes:

> [Caregiving] is like flowing into a fast-moving river. I was so busy trying to navigate the swirling, rapid currents,

1. Hoblitzelle, *Ten Thousand Joys and Ten Thousand Sorrows: A Couple's Journey Through Alzheimer's*.

I would forget the magnitude of what we were dealing with. Much of it was invisible. The psychic toll was the hardest. I needed to be aware all the time. I lived on the edge of the moment, always awaiting the next gap.[2]

Every moment with Earl, day and night, I am in a heightened awareness. My job is to be finely tuned to his world. I need to be open to receive and respond to anything, no matter how tired I may be or how I feel. And sometimes I fail. Hoblitzelle again:

> I lived in constant challenge. I needed to patrol my own personal boundaries so I didn't lose myself in being his indispensable other, yet simultaneously I had to remain receptive and accepting of those intrusions of his psychic need.[3]

I live in several worlds at once. There is Earl's world and the complexities of his disease. There is my world, apart from his. There is our friends' and families' worlds, and the world at large.

Here is an example of something that is hard for me as a twenty-four hour, seven days per week, care partner: the local bank we use has been sold to another bank, which means I need to change our routing numbers. I need to contact businesses to tell them our new debit card numbers. I need to order new checks. These are the kinds of tasks that send me over the edge. I often wonder if I have energy for anything outside of our home. Banking is not something I can delegate to someone else. As a care partner, this is the sort of aggravation that pushes me over the edge.

However, any situation can be a source of growth, right? Although I sputter and flail at times, I have mostly found equilibrium as a care partner, at least for now. This is made easier because of Earl's ability to be vulnerable: he lets me help him.

I'm trying to think of taking care of Earl as a meditation—a practice of patience, generosity, discipline, contemplation, and wisdom. I work on seeing things as opportunities. I mean, we can

---

2. Hoblitzelle, *Ten Thousand Joys and Ten Thousand Sorrows*, 9.
3. Hoblitzelle, *Ten Thousand Joys and Ten Thousand Sorrows*, 83.

both be miserable, or I can respond to Earl with love. How I respond can either make or break our day.

When Earl is tucked into bed, I read to him, and then offer a breathing exercise: "With your eyes closed, breathe in. Now, breathe out." I repeat this simple exercise for five to ten minutes. Earl loves this practice and I am so glad! We both find it a restful and meaningful way to end the day.

Last night, I shared with Earl a meditation from Richard Rohr. One paragraph especially spoke to both of us. (My thanks to Tara, also a care partner, for sending this meditation to us):

> While change can force a transformation, spiritual transformation always includes a disconcerting reorientation. It can either help people to find new meaning or it can force people to close down and slowly turn bitter. The difference is determined precisely by the quality of our inner life, our practices, and our spirituality.[4]

Earl and I find ourselves on an "unexpected shore." The landscape is always changing, and I must remain vigilant. This vigilance—the constant need to reorient—best describes what care-partnering is like for me.

We had another meaningful conversation recently when Lewy took a vacation. We talked about the extraordinary year we have had and what it has meant to both of us.

Earl said he knew he would need help walking eventually. I said he might need help in the bathroom also. He balked at that; he said he would not like that to happen. He reiterated that he doesn't want either of us to suffer. I asked him if it came to a point where he couldn't eat or drink by himself, would he want to stop eating and drinking? He said he didn't think so, that he would prefer hospice care.

He asked me what would happen to him if I died first, then he smiled and said he figured Jen, Rich, and I had a plan. That seemed to comfort him.

4. Rohr, *The Wisdom Pattern*, 83-84.

Then he told me he was looking forward to death when it comes. He said he doesn't fear it, and how helpful it is that we can talk about his dying. Earl said someday we would unite on the other side, which brought tears to both of our eyes, and then a tight hug.

May these words remind me—and all of us—that love can face even dying with honesty and grace.

Love,
Juanita

September 14, 2020

Dear Family and Friends,

What do you suppose Earl gave me as a wedding present the night before we married in 1965? Jewelry, perhaps? Maybe a favorite book or a much-loved object he treasured? No, his gift was a set of leather-bound encyclopedias. He purchased the set with the compensation he received tutoring Missouri University football players in mathematics.

In Earl's teens and early twenties, he read every single page of the *Encyclopedia Britannica*—every volume, from A to Z. He wanted me to have the same opportunity. Holy moly! His gift quickly informed me that Earl's gift-giving might miss the mark from time to time.

How often do any of us miss the mark on how to best relate to our loved one? I don't know about you, but I probably spent way too many years responding to Earl with a "love language" that resonated with me rather than with him. I've come to understand why I was consistently disappointed that Earl didn't give me words of affirmation: it wasn't his "love language," and he didn't know it was mine. I guess I assumed he would read my mind and figure it out. How silly.

You know how exciting it is when you find just the right book? The one with countless marked-up pages? In August, I found that book for just this time in our lives: *Keeping Love Alive as Memories Fade: The Five Love Languages.*[1] The authors

---

1. Chapman et al., *Keeping Love Alive as Memories Fade: The Five Love Languages*.

describe how loving someone with dementia becomes a one-way street. Our loved one's ability to show love is compromised, yet research confirms that the emotional life of someone with dementia is alive.[2] How I respond to Earl is critical. I want to induce positive feelings as much as possible.

When I was a counselor in private practice, I sometimes suggested couples read Chapman's book *The Five Love Languages*.[3] Although there is scientific criticism of Chapman's work, which centers on a lack of empirical evidence, I believe the concepts, under the right circumstances, can be useful.

According to Chapman, the Five Love Languages are: words of affirmation, quality time, gifts, acts of service, and physical touch.[4]

Chapman and his colleagues suggest that all five languages are important to each of us, but one or two will stand out from the rest.[5] Because Earl is no longer able to take the quiz himself, the book instructed me to take the quiz first, and then take it for Earl, imagining how he would answer the questions.

What I discovered absolutely delights me: Earl has two languages, equal in importance. They are quality time and touch. It confirms why Earl wants me to watch TV with him (something I don't always want to do): he perceives it as quality time. He loves watching comedies with me. It also confirms why he recently told me the happiest time of his life was last February, when Rich visited and our family was all together.

His language of touch explains why he likes to sit on the couch together and hold hands or rub my feet. Why he likes cheek kisses at night when I tuck him in, and morning hugs. These were all things I was already doing, perhaps intuiting their importance from his responses. But it was validating to recognize these are, indeed, his love languages. (Love languages may change

2. Chapman et al., *Keeping Love Alive.*

3. Chapman, *The Five Love Languages: How to Express Heartfelt Commitment to Your Mate.*

4. Chapman, *The Five Love Languages.*

5. Chapman et al., *Keeping Love Alive.*

with the progression of dementia, so I will need to keep alert for that possibility.[6])

Equally revealing was relearning what my love languages are. The authors emphasize the importance of care partners knowing their "languages," to try to keep their bucket at least half full.[7] As a caregiver, it is easy to feel depleted. Or, as a friend who is caregiving recently said to me, "All color has disappeared from my life."

Like Earl, I have two languages with equal value. They are words of affirmation and quality time. This helps me understand one of the reasons I share these updates. Some of you send me a response. Your words are affirming and help me fill my bucket. Apparently, I benefit from having cheerleaders. I receive cards from friends, which is also affirming. Rich and Jen are both really good at affirming me and the care I give their dad. Perhaps they have intuited it is my "language." With this knowledge, I can specifically ask friends for affirmation.

My other "language," quality time, is harder for me to experience presently. I greatly miss in-depth conversations with friends. Earl and I still experience quality time when Lewy is absent.

I will be able to offer Earl better care, and more love, understanding what his "languages" are. And, I know what I need to ask for from family and friends to keep my bucket from being empty. Thus, this treasure of a book has offered both of us another avenue forward on the journey no one wants to take.

Stay safe and love well,
Juanita

---

6. Chapman et al., *Keeping Love Alive.*

7. Chapman et al., *Keeping Love Alive.*

December 29, 2020

Dear Friends and Family,

Thank you to those who support and remember us in so many ways. You put a smile on Earl's face when I tell him we have heard from you. You lift our spirits when you offer reminders we are not alone. During these hard days, let's all be asking each other, "Are you okay?"—and then really listening to the response.

We haven't had Christmas lights or a tree inside our home since Earl's diagnosis. The inside lights can intensify hallucinations. Instead, our home has been filled with flowers.

In late November, Earl began to ask me about stringing holiday lights outside, as he had always done around our homes. He loved the sparkle of the outside lights. He said they welcomed people to our home. Unfortunately, we didn't have a functional outside power outlet, so there was no way we could have lights outside. I didn't know how to explain this to Earl.

I shared my frustration and sorrow that I couldn't make the lights happen, by text, with my book group. My friends, the elves, went to work. One of the members said she knew an electrician who could install an outlet on our front porch in the next few weeks. This lovely group of women collectively paid for the installation. I felt deep gratitude.

Thus, Earl was able to string lights on a bush in our front yard. I took a photo to capture the image, through my tears, to share with our real-life elves: the electrician and the book group.

Every night, before going to bed, Earl opens the front door to admire his lights.

If we look for them, there are always tiny graces—small, overlooked moments, even in the darkest of times.

It's curious the paths journal-writing takes me on. For the past month, I've been writing about my mother's relationship to caregiving. My mom cared for her mother, her brother, and her husband, all at different times in her later years. She cared for each of them in her home until their deaths. I no longer lived at home during these times, and she seldom spoke to me about what offering care was like, or whether it took a toll on her.

Did I learn some things about offering care from my mom? From her steadiness, her quiet nature, her devotion to family? Did she model for me something I hoped I would never need?

Although Mom died when I was in my thirties, she has been a guide for me this past month as I figure out how to move forward as a care partner.

With the help of the book *The Five Invitations: Discovering What Death Can Teach Us About Living*, whose author, Frank Ostaseski, is a Zen Buddhist, I've been observing the difference between "surface mind" and "calm depths."[1] When I'm in surface mind, all I can do is react. The author writes, "It's as though you are at the total mercy of the storm, you're in a tiny rowboat in a wild sea. When you travel into the calm depths, you can act from a place of wisdom and compassion."[2] This is the place my mother modeled: a deep, calm presence.

The philosopher Blaise Pascal writes, "I have often said that the sole cause of man's unhappiness is that he doesn't know how to stay quietly in his room."[3]

At night, after I tuck Earl in, read to him, and guide him in our breathing exercise, I retreat to my own room to journal and rest. The quiet of writing helps me plumb new depths. I somehow

1. Ostaseski, *The Five Invitations*.
2. Ostaseski, *The Five Invitations*, 194.
3. Pascal, *Pensées*, 43.

feel protected. I can't really explain why I feel protected, but there is something about the depths I travel to in my writing. The deeper I explore, the more expansive I become. I can allow thoughts, feelings, and ideas to come and go without being swept away by any of them. It is this time, journaling alone at night, that keeps me going. The writing allows me to fiercely love this wonderful, gentle man who is fading away before my eyes.

My daily goal is to create a safe refuge for Earl. I believe the slow pace of our current life, and my consistency in being available to him, helps him trust me and feel secure. We live one day at a time with intention, gratitude, and naps. We rest in the quiet.

Out of nowhere, Earl told me that he would like for me to find a choral group to sing with, like I used to do many years ago. He said I could leave him alone and if he fell, "Well, so what?" I told him I thought it would be a year before there were singing groups again, due to the pandemic. He replied, "I'm not sure I'll be here in a year."

Be safe, be kind, and take good care,
Juanita

P.S. The current bedtime book I'm reading to Earl is *Hometown Tales: Reflections of Kindness, Peace, and Joy* by the Quaker, Philip Gulley.[4] I just finished listening to the immensely enjoyable audiobook *Greenlights*, read by its author.[5] We've been enjoying Harry Chapin's music, especially the song "Circle."[6]

P.P.S. Consider renting *Robin's Wish* on a streaming service.[7] The documentary offers a moving portrayal of beloved actor and comedian Robin Williams' last years living with Lewy body dementia, which was sadly misdiagnosed and never appropriately treated.

4. Gulley, *Hometown Tales*.
5. McConaughey, *Greenlights*.
6. Chapin, "Circle," *Sniper and Other Love Songs*.
7. *Robin's Wish*, directed by Tyler Norwood.

February 2, 2021

Dear Friends and Family,

We are all weary from the Covid pandemic, aren't we? Some of you have been ill, some of you have had a loved one die. Many people I have had contact with feel lonely and are grieving what has been lost. We all are in a mess, hoping that before too long we can resume a somewhat normal life.

With empathy for all of you and what we are all enduring, I share with you what life has been like for Earl and me the past couple of months.

Almost every morning, when Earl is ready to start his day, he asks for oatmeal and an orange cut into tiny slices. I've recently become more mindful that fixing his breakfast is a daily nurturing ritual. As I stir his oatmeal, I stand at the kitchen window, where I can watch the birds at our bird feeders. It's all quite soothing. The stirring reminds me of a passage from *We* by Robert Johnson:

> Stirring the oatmeal is a humble act—not exciting or thrilling. But it symbolizes a relatedness that brings love down to earth. It represents a willingness to share ordinary human life, to find meaning in the simple unromantic tasks, earning a living, living within a budget, and putting out the garbage. To "stir the oatmeal" means to find the relatedness, the value, even the beauty, in simple and ordinary things, not to eternally demand a cosmic drama, an entertainment, or an extraordinary intensity to everything. It represents the discovery of the sacred in the midst of the humble and the ordinary.[1]

1. Johnson, *We: Understanding the Psychology of Romantic Love*, 89.

My life with Earl, as he slips away cognitively and physically, has become sacred in our ordinary life. I'm becoming better at anticipating what makes him comfortable. He can still chuckle when we manage to put his clothes on backwards.

But in truth, there is less of him to share. He frequently loses words or can't finish a sentence. Often, he tells me he is confused. He depends on me to keep him safe. He knows I love him.

Where once we would have had conversation, Earl and I sit next to each other in silence, or listen to music or an audiobook, holding hands. Occasionally, I'll reach up and touch his face. He smiles, and his blue eyes glisten. The feeling of love is tender in the room. There is sadness and joy between us: the fullness of our relationship.

I'd be in a far different place if I wasn't able to carve out alonetime in the evening and early morning. I haven't had any respite for over a year. Caring for myself while he sleeps is my key to being loving and patient when he is awake.

But most of all, it is Earl's disposition, his gentleness, his kindness, that helps me "stir his oatmeal" with good spirits. I am in awe at how he accepts his disease with such good grace.

> *May you feel safe*
> *May you feel healthy*
> *May you feel happy*
> *May you feel at ease.*
> —Metta meditation of loving-kindness[2]

Love,
Juanita

P.S. *Recipes for a Sacred Life* by Rivvy Neshama[3] is my current bedtime reading to Earl. We are listening to the audiobook *Owls of the Eastern Ice*, read by its author, Jonathan Slaght.[4] Earl and

---

2. Variation of "Metta Meditation," *Lion's Roar.*

3. Neshama, *Recipes for a Sacred Life: True Stories and Few Miracles.*

4. Slaght, *Owls of the Eastern Ice: A Quest to Find and Save the World's Largest Owl.*

I are also listening to chapters from *Vesper Flights*, stories of bird behaviors, read by its English author, Helen MacDonald, who also wrote the magnificent book *H is for Hawk*.[5] (I've listened to *Vesper Flights* twice while doing jigsaw puzzles on my iPad.)

P.P.S. I've had both of my Covid-19 vaccine shots. Earl gets his first one today. Hooray!

---

5. MacDonald, *Vesper Flights* and *H is for Hawk*.

March 17, 2021

I'm weary and feeling the weight of being a care partner.

The kind and practical VA nurse suggested that, after Earl is vaccinated, he might benefit from speech therapy and PT for movement therapy. When she suggested this, I felt a knot in my chest. Am I doing right by Earl, by not encouraging him to seek these therapies? But Earl has been clear: no unnecessary treatments. He does not want any therapies that might prolong his life.

Most of the time, it is easy for me to communicate his wishes. The many conversations Earl and I have had help me be firm in how I reply. But still, there is a moment when I do hesitate, especially if I sense a negative vibe from the nurse.

I remind myself: this is Earl's body, his life, his choosing. My role is not to manage him, but to walk with him.

In February, we were watching the Super Bowl together, something Earl and I had been looking forward to, when Earl abruptly turned off the TV. He complained the referees were not doing their jobs. He proceeded to go to bed, sulking, still wearing his day clothes.

I had prepared our favorite Super Bowl food and had been looking forward to a few hours of normalcy. Instead, I was left by myself in the quiet. I didn't dare turn on the TV back on, because even if I muted the sound, the flashing lights can agitate Earl. I sat on the couch in the living room, in the dark, and cried. I am so tired of the endless grind of holding everything together.

I have written email updates about the REM sleep and the violent behavior that would sometimes occur. I'm not sure I captured the raw terror I felt. How scary it was when Earl pushed me out of bed with his strong legs, pulled my hair so that my scalp ached for days, or put a pillow over my face. How do you begin to describe that?

I moved to a different bed to sleep. I could have done it sooner. In hindsight I sure wish I had.

And here is something I should write: when I described these REM sleep behaviors to the VA social worker, the fall/panic button they ordered for us was to use *when I felt unsafe*, as well as for Earl's falls.

There have been times when a friend has visited and Earl chats for a while, and then abruptly stands up. He says something like, "This no longer interests me," and leaves the room. I apologize and feel embarrassed. I am certain his friends understand, yet it sure feels awkward and inhospitable. When it happens, I always find Earl curled up on the small couch in the TV room, quite agitated. I check on him gently and then leave him alone to cool off, while I cool off, too.

Boy, do I need strength tonight!

The Late Stage: February to May 2021

Daily Rhythms of Care

"Love is how you stay alive, even after you are gone."
—Mitch Albom, *Tuesdays with Morrie.*[1]

Our rhythms have unraveled. Earl no longer follows a clock. I still rise early. I'm showered and dressed by 7:00 AM out of habit more than need. Some mornings, Earl wakes around 8:00 AM. Other days, he sleeps until mid-afternoon. His body follows its own mysterious tides now.

He sleeps in a hospital bed provided by the VA. This is a gift that has made caring for him so much easier; now I don't need to bend to reach him. By adjusting the head of the bed, I can sit him up to eat. I found a rolling tray-table that adjusts to the perfect height. It delights Earl to sit in bed and eat meals on his tray. I'm certain it is his current favorite activity. When he wakes, whether it's 10:00 AM or 3:00 PM, I ask him if he is hungry. He replies, "I would like to have breakfast in bed, served on the tray." It seems to really tickle him to be able to eat in bed. To see him enjoy himself, with such a simple request, lightens my heart.

---

1. Albom, *Tuesdays with Morrie*, 133.

If he asks, I help him change clothes. Sometimes he wants to; often he doesn't. Dressing has become a delicate negotiation. I follow his lead.

He still uses the bathroom on his own, with only two accidents so far. I installed a bidet after reading how helpful it could be. Unfortunately, Earl just finds it confusing. The bidet may have been helpful if it had been installed much earlier.

Earl continues to reach for his electric razor, though he says it's broken. We have three—none of them faulty—but he can no longer make sense of them. I do my best to help, having watched videos on how to shave him gently. I'm not good at it at all.

His appetite flickers like a candle—sometimes strong, sometimes barely present. I cook what I know he loves, but more often than not, I end up scraping full plates into the bin. I try not to let this waste of food, and this uncertain part of his LBD, undo me.

Showering is rare. Instead, I use specially designed bath cloths, warmed and moistened, and sing softly as I clean his body. He doesn't like this, but tolerates it when I sing.

Toothbrushing is symbolic now—just a few swipes. He doesn't let me help, but he does allow me to offer him mouthwash.

I'm no longer able to sleep well at night, even in my separate room. Earl is restless. I'm always listening for him to wake up. If he tries to get out of bed by himself, he is likely to fall. I get up and check on him every time I hear him move in his bed. He is also keenly aware of any movements I make. If I get out of bed for any reason, he seems to have supersonic radar, knowing I'm up. It is becoming nearly impossible to get any rest.

With no schedule I can count on, I feel unmoored.

But one thing helps: the unobtrusive little cameras the VA provided. Since Earl cannot be left alone, if he is in bed sleeping and I need to step outside to just have a moment or breathe some fresh air, I coordinate with my daughter. She can keep a watch on the cameras via her phone, from her home next door, even when she's working. If Earl stirs while I'm outside, Jen comes right over, or texts me to go back inside. It's a system that gives me just enough freedom to keep going.

Even without a clear routine, one ritual remains. At bedtime—no matter what the day has brought—I sit by Earl's bed. I read aloud a short passage or story, then we breathe together. *In. Out. In, and out.* He closes his eyes to the rhythm of my voice, to the breath we share. After he's asleep, I kiss his cheek and tell him, "I'll see you in the morning light." This has not changed. And I am grateful.

April 5, 2021

Dear Friends and Family,

This update will provide you with a glimpse of our life right now. The Durham VA has offered us eleven hours of overnight respite per week from a home-care agency. Earl told the program supervisor that I was exhausted. He agreed that we need someone who can watch him if he wakes and moves around the house. However, later he said, "To be clear, I would like the overnight help to be my daughter." So, we shall see how easily he will accept someone he doesn't know into our home.

The VA has a coach program, which is home-based dementia care. It consists of a nurse and a social worker who come to our home once a month. Due to Covid-19, we have not had very much in-person contact, which is a disappointment, because I find their visits uplifting.

On April ninth, on one of their in-person visits, the nurse gave Earl a cognitive test while I visited with the social worker in another room. A year and a half ago, Earl scored twenty-one (mild dementia). Today he scored eight (severe dementia). I cried when the nurse told me the results. It was a shock because Earl and I still occasionally have meaningful conversations. She said Earl would be in very bad shape, with little reality, if it weren't for my "exceptional care."

The nurse also said how unusual Earl is. "His kindness and thoughtful attitude to LBD is remarkable." She asked him if he was sad, angry, or depressed. He told her, "My son and daughter make me happy. I have a grandson who is becoming a fine young man. My son-in-law is a wonderful father. Juanita is my teammate. Why should I be unhappy?" The nurse said his attitude was astounding.

The social worker is concerned that I have very little emotional support or opportunities to be with friends. Now that my friends are vaccinated, they are going places with each other again. I cried and shared how left out—and left behind—I feel. He asked me if I felt resentful or depressed. I could honestly answer no. Just sad.

The social worker asked me if there were troubling behaviors with Earl. Of course there are, but I told him I could usually see the cause and knew how to prevent most of these situations. The social worker said it's likely because I've been willing to learn how to manage Lewy, that Earl doesn't have a lot of troubling behaviors. A part of me believes that, but I also believe some of it is just luck, and some is Earl's mostly pleasant disposition that stems from his many years of spiritual work.

When the four of us came back into the same room—nurse, social worker, Earl, and I—I made sure to repeat Earl's wishes that he did not want to extend his life. Both the nurse and social worker said they could support that decision. They told me to be sure Earl's primary care provider signed the Medical Orders for Scope of Treatment (MOST) form.

Before the two of them left, they told us again that we were unusual in our acceptance of Earl's diagnosis, and the care and respect that was evident between us. They said they wished there was a way to share our journey with others. They said that many of the families they work with are in denial about the diagnosis and therefore don't educate themselves about LBD.

I loved having them in our home. I can't wait until they return in a month. The empathy and positive affirmation they share with us, helps us both.

In loving Earl through dementia, I have been stretched into strength I never knew I had.

This quote says it all: "Darkness deserves gratitude. It is the alleluia point at which we learn to understand that all growth does not take place in the sunlight."[1]

Thank you for being on this journey with us,
Juanita

1. Chittister and Williams, *Uncommon Gratitude: Alleluia for All That Is*, 185.

April 28, 2021

Dear Family and Friends,

Happy spring! Here in North Carolina, the azaleas are starting to bloom, tulips and irises are popping open, and the spectacular spring-flowering trees are likely to take your breath away.

Grandson Sam and I are fully vaccinated, so we can bake bread together again! Honestly, I hadn't realized how terribly I missed this, and what a boost it would be to be kneading dough side by side. The conversation is easy and the laughs come often.

Jen is once again able to spend time with her dad, and we anticipate a visit from Rich as soon as he can get vaccinated. Hugs and tears, what joy!

With Earl sleeping so much during the day, I decided to sign up for an online photography course. I've never been interested in taking anything but rudimentary photos, but I'm fascinated by photos others have taken. In the course, every week we are given a new topic and encouraged to share photos on the topic. One of my favorite topics was "reflection and action." I find that I percolate for much of the week before taking and posting my photos. Others' pictures intrigue me. I ponder how they reflect the week's topic. The practice has opened my eyes to what may be hidden in a photo, and yet right there when you look with a new perspective. I've been introduced to a larger world, right here in my living room. Even with my life narrowing and routines fixed, I have found a new way of stimulating my mind.

The book *Effortless Beauty: Photography as an Expression of Eye, Mind, and Heart* has also inspired me to see the world with new-old-eyes.[1] Its author writes:

> You are aligned with your heart and mind, your being, your intention with the present moment, and what is waiting to come forth. It's true whether you are writing a song, writing a book, telling a story, or taking a photograph, it's a three-way conference call between what is being expressed, the present moment, and our heart-mind connection.[2]

Interestingly, the practice of mindfully taking photos has also helped me stay in the present moment with Earl. I see more beauty around us and in him. I read somewhere the importance of taking heaps of photos of someone who is failing, as someday you will wish you had more pictures. Sunday, I took a picture of Earl "reading" the Sunday comics. He quite enjoyed the feel of holding the paper, and I have a photo of his delight.

Life in our home is challenging for both of us. A good-natured Earl needs a lot of help. I'm pretty good at some tasks and lousy at others. More days than not, I realize how much my role has changed. A dear friend once told me she went from lover, to friend, to nurse, in caring for her ailing husband. I'm definitely in the nurse stage. I'm constantly adapting and learning new skills to try to keep up.

People with Lewy typically sleep a lot as the disease progresses. There are days when Earl sleeps until 3:00 PM. As a care partner, one might see that as a blessing, as time to relax or regroup. The problem is, I never know how long he will sleep. He can awaken at 7:00 AM, 3:00 PM, or any time in between. There is no way to predict what the day will bring. The not-knowing keeps me on pins and needles.

1. DuBose, *Effortless Beauty: Photography as an Expression of Eye, Mind, and Heart*.

2. DuBose, *Effortless Beauty: Photography as an Expression of Eye, Mind, and Heart*, unpaginated.

Nights are the most difficult. Or maybe it's the lack of sleep adding up. All night, I listen for Earl stirring in his bed—night is when he is most likely to fall. And his radar persists: if he hears me go to the bathroom or get a glass of water, he calls for me. He invariably wants me to sit by his side.

The VA approved night-time care to help me get some rest. My hopes soared when I met with the manager of the home-care agency last week. She vetted us and immediately put us on their schedule. Every night, I leave the porch light on, looking forward to meeting the home-care helper who is scheduled to arrive. Every night, I think, "Tonight, I will be able to sink into bed, knowing someone else is looking out for Earl." For five nights in a row, no one has come. I wait, hour by hour. It adds to my exhaustion. When I called the agency, they said, "Unfortunately, this happens. Sometimes aides don't show up." My hopes are dashed. Should I keep leaving the porch light on?

For now, I'm doing my very best to be content to love, encourage, and appreciate Earl in our home. I try to constantly evaluate my physical, mental, emotional, and spiritual states. I'm so very tired. But I work at being comfortable with our life as it is. Meditation, journaling, napping when Earl sleeps, and our night-time reading and breathing practices truly help.

Every day, I can find a smidgen of joy, and every day, I experience deep sadness. "The deeper that sorrow carves into your being, the more joy you can contain," writes Kahlil Gibran in *The Prophet*.[3] My heart is trying to find space for all this.

In the evening, when I tuck Earl into bed, he asks me what I'm going to read to him. No matter what the struggles of the day were, this is our time of "ritual," of slow breaths, of tenderness. I feel such gratitude for the precious time we have together.

So my friends, farewell for now,
Juanita

3. Gibran, *The Prophet*, 51.

P.S. What I'm currently reading to Earl at bedtime: *Living Buddha, Living Christ.*[4]

P.P.S. Audiobooks I've been listening to while doing jigsaw puzzles on my iPad: *The Children's Blizzard*[5] and *Calypso*, read by its author.[6] Earl and I have been listening to the music of The Limelighters[7] and *World Hits on Harmonica*.[8] Earl loves listening to artists who play the harmonica.

P.P.P.S. We received the research results from the study Earl participated in. Some of you will recall that Earl participated in a study at NCSU in 2019, shortly after he was diagnosed with LBD.[9] The research question was, "Does depression interact with cognitive ability in impaired older adults to predict motivation to engage in cognitively demanding activities?" Basically, the study found that people who have mild cognitive problems and who are not depressed do better as the cognitive symptoms grow more severe. Being depressed exacerbates cognitive decline. The study also found that people with mild cognitive decline who were not depressed were just as happy, or happier, than those with no cognitive issues.

4. Thich Nhat Hanh, *Living Buddha, Living Christ.*

5. Benjamin, *The Children's Blizzard.*

6. Sedaris, *Calypso.*

7. The Limelighters, *Joy Across the Land.*

8. Rademakers, *World Hits on Harmonia.*

9. Neupert et al., "Analysis of Cognitive Engagement."

May 10, 2021

Yesterday was Mother's Day. Earl complained of discomfort in his stomach, which is very unusual for him. He asked if Noah could come check on him, which Noah always gladly does. I knew Earl wanted reassurance. Noah provided it. I kept a close watch of Earl all day.

In the evening, after I finished reading to him, he said he needed to go to the bathroom. This has seldom happened after he is tucked in. He got out of bed and leaned against a nearby wall. Before I could get to him, he fell. My gut knew something was different this time.

I wear a simple, slender necklace which has a small charm. It looks like a normal necklace. On the back of the charm is a button. Pressing the button alerts my emergency contacts: my daughter, son, and son-in-law. I wear the necklace because it is an easy way to alert my family that I need help, without using a phone. (Phone calls disturb Earl.) I have never needed to use the button before. I pressed the button. Within minutes, my daughter and son-in-law let themselves in. My son in Oregon asked to be included in the emergency contacts, so he knows to text me.

Noah was able to get Earl back into his bed. Earl seemed unusually agitated. I think we all knew something was off.

Jen and Noah stayed with me. Earl fell again at 3:00 AM. Noah could not get Earl up this time. I called EMS for a "fall assist." After picking him up, the medics suggested they transport Earl to the hospital. I replied with an emphatic, "*No.*" I know Earl does not want life-extending care.

Early this morning, after Jen and Noah had gone home to get ready for work, I got a text from Jen: "Noah thinks it's time to contact hospice."

I was relieved. I didn't know I would feel such relief—to be told to contact hospice. I'm incredibly grateful for Noah's good sense and clarity. I was overwhelmed and needed guidance.

I called the VA nurse who has visited us several times. I told her we need hospice assistance.

"Okay. I will put the order into the computer. One of the local hospices will contact you."

"Will they really? How long will it take?"

"Very quickly. Why do you ask?"

I sigh. Is there a word that goes beyond exhaustion? "I ask because the night-care person the VA promised has never shown up."

This seemed to distress her. She assured me hospice would call. And within minutes, my phone buzzed. It was the manager of a regional, for-profit hospice company, who would be sending someone over in two hours.

Jen was with me when the hospice representative arrived. We were expecting compassion and comfort. Instead, he acted like a used-car salesman. He had a briefcase and a clipboard. He listed symptoms, checking them off on his clipboard like we were talking about car-repair problems. He said, "Well, I'm not sure your husband will qualify. I need to ask my supervisor."

Jen and I just looked at each other when he left. We were nearly speechless. I knew this wouldn't do. Where was the empathy? This was like a sales transaction—and a bad one at that.

I immediately contacted Earl's neurologist, who is affiliated with both the VA and Duke. I told him we need Duke Hospice—specifically Duke Hospice. Duke Hospice called within minutes. They said they would come first thing the next morning. We knew it might be a long night, but Jen and I agreed it would be worth the wait.

As promised, the next morning, the Duke Hospice social worker came. She sat with Jen and me. There was no clipboard. There was no checklist of symptoms or doubt about Earl qualifying. Her very first question was, "Tell me your love story. How did you and Earl meet?"

The contrast between the two hospices was extraordinary. Jen and I were so stunned that we felt like we needed to double-check—we asked if Earl qualified. Of course he did.

Duke Hospice set up a care schedule and said they would send a box of medications through the mail. They do this for all new hospice families to have on hand. We are supposed to keep it in the refrigerator; that's where all hospice families keep it, so hospice workers always know where to find it.

Several hours later, Duke Hospice personnel arrived to begin offering care to Earl.

May 14, 2021

Last night was a terrible night. Not just terrible, but traumatic.

Earl was agitated, could not sleep, would not settle, would not stay in bed. He had never been like this before. I used the button on my necklace, for the second time, and Jen and Noah immediately came over. While they were with Earl, I quietly called the on-call hospice night nurse for guidance. She was calm and soothing. She said I needed the medication that was in the hospice box. It had not yet arrived in the mail. It had only been a short time—and this week there has been a nation-wide pharmacy and delivery slow-down, due to Covid.

This meant I would need to go to the all-night Walgreens at 1 AM. The pharmacy was thirty minutes away.

The night hospice nurse told me I could call as often as I wanted to throughout the night. Giving Earl new medications had risks. Her empathy and knowledge of LBD was very reassuring.

My daughter went to get the medicine. Noah stayed to help me manage Earl, who was so agitated I was scared what might happen.

Because Earl had complained about his stomach hurting a few days before (which was most unusual), I suspected he had an infection. I had read enough about LBD symptoms to suspect he might have a urinary tract infection. I also knew he would not want treatment for this, or any, infection. But what was happening was terrifying. He was in constant motion. He was agitated. I felt helpless.

When Jen returned with the medication, she and I stood at the kitchen sink and said a silent prayer that the medicine would help Earl. What if it made his agitation worse? This was a 50% probability with LBD.

Everything Earl was doing was so out of character. I was beside myself with fear and worry. Eventually, the medicine worked. Earl was able to rest. Jen rolled out a yoga mat and spent what was left of the night on the floor next to her dad's bed.

The whole night was bizarre—unreal. It was scary and exhausting. I knew there was no way I could manage Earl at home any longer. Not if this was the new norm.

The next morning, we made a plan to transfer Earl to the Duke Hospice facility.

May 16, 2021

Dear All,

Two weeks ago, Earl and I sat side by side on our living room couch. I asked him if he would like for me to read letters to him. I had organized an album of all the correspondence he had written or received since we first met in 1963. I had the brilliant idea to use the voice-recorder app on my phone while I read him snippets of letters: letters he wrote to me, to his mom, to his children; and letters he received, one from my dad, others from his students, his friends, his children. As I shared letters with him, he shared memories with me. We did this for forty-five minutes. It was one of the rare times lately that Lewy was not messing with his cognition.

I took advantage of Lewy being absent, turned to him, and asked him how he was currently feeling about dying. In just above a whisper, as he was losing volume in his voice, he told me he was not afraid to die. Looking at me with great love in his blue eyes, he said, "I just don't want to be separated from you." Holding hands, we talked about the fact we would only be separated physically. He concluded the conversation by saying he hoped his physical journey could end in the care of hospice.

Today, two weeks after that unforgettable conversation, Earl is completely bedridden and in the care of Duke Hospice. He is dying.

The two and a half years since his official diagnosis have been an unexpected gift for Earl and me. Even within Lewy's never-ending tempest, our love has deepened. We have experienced the raw, vulnerable parts of loving under very trying conditions.

We, his family, are at peace. Jen, Rich, Noah, and Sam have showered him with love and respect. Our hearts are clear.

Some tips I've learned:

- No two hospices are alike. They can be as different as night and day. It's okay to shop for the right one.

- If someone in your family is considering long-term care insurance, consider a linked-benefit policy, which offers dual protection for long-term care coverage and a death benefit for beneficiaries.

- Use the voice recorder app on your phone or tablet. Ask questions of your loved ones. Tell stories and preserve the recording.

- The old cliche, "Hold those you love close, and imagine this is the last day you will have with them" is true. Love fiercely.

Breathing in, breathing out,
Juanita

June 30, 2021

Dear Friends and Family,

Because I find writing therapeutic, I will continue to send you updates, even though Earl died on May eighteenth.

We moved Earl from our home to the Duke Hospice facility, Hock Pavilion, four days before he died, as he needed more care than we could manage at home.

The hospice facility was lovely. Each room had a small outside area, with big windows and a glass door. The hospital bed could be wheeled to this private patio if a patient wanted to be outside.

My daughter and I met with the hospice doctor, who was forthright and provided helpful assurances. The doctor told us it is rare for a family to all be aligned when the patient has elected for no treatment. (We had very little opportunity to interact with the hospice social worker and chaplain who were assigned to us, because Earl declined so quickly. Jen and I visited by speaker phone with both of them. We were certain we would have enjoyed a relationship with them, had there been more time to get acquainted.)

As I sat at Earl's bedside, he reached for my hands. Not just one, but both. His grip was fierce, as if holding my hands anchored him. Words felt unnecessary, though I knew hearing is the last sense to fade. What mattered was the silent language between us, the deep communion of our souls, carried through touch. In that clasp, I knew this was his final love language.

"Have you finished your rituals? I am ready to leave." These were the last words Earl spoke to me, the day before he died. His words did not surprise me. He knew how important creating meaningful rituals was to me. Somehow it made sense he would ask me if they were finished, for then he could leave. There was a sweetness to his words—a communication between the two of us that only we would understand.

Earl had a peaceful death, witnessed by his son. Rich had spent the night sitting at his dad's bedside, talking to him, touching him, and softly playing music. At 4:20 AM, his dad simply stopped breathing. Rich immediately called Jen and me; we had gone home to rest. We jumped into the car and quickly joined Rich.

With Earl's body present, my children and I shared in a poignant goodbye ritual. Through our tears, we blessed each part of Earl. As we said each blessing, we laid our hands on the corresponding part of Earl's body.

> We bless your head, and your mind. We thank you for the words, thoughts, and ideas that have influenced our lives.
>
> We bless your eyes, that have looked on us with such love.
>
> We bless your ears, for the way you listened to us, and to your inner world.
>
> We bless your heart, for the love you have so generously given.
>
> We bless your hands, that helped us and cared for us and so many others.
>
> We bless your legs and feet, for all the ways they have taken you on journeys throughout this life.

After we finished blessing his body, the three of us lingered quietly for a while. It hit me hard—it would be the last time the four of us would be in the same room together.

Noah and Sam then visited (Covid protocols limited how many could be in the room at one time). We were not rushed by hospice staff and spent quality time saying goodbye. I hugged my grandson and told him his grandfather had had a good death.

I believe, but will never know for certain, that Earl had developed an acute infection, one which probably could have been treated with a hospital stay and medications.

Why anyone with Lewy body dementia would want to extend their life is beyond my comprehension. Often it is someone within the family who wants their loved one treated: out of loyalty, fear of being left alone, or fear of death. Fortunately, from Earl's first visit with his primary care practitioner, he had clearly stated, "I only want comfort care." He documented his wishes legally and kept a DNR (Do Not Resuscitate) card on him even though he never left our home.

None of us in his family hesitated in following through with what he wanted. When I spoke with his doctors and told them Earl would be moving to the hospice facility, they suggested Earl be taken to the ER for treatment instead. Fortunately, when I replied no, Earl wanted no treatment, I received no pushback from his doctors. They were respectful and understanding, because Earl and I had been consistent in stating what he wanted.

We, his family, were clear-hearted and clear-headed. We knew exactly what Earl wanted. He had told us he did not fear death.

Earl gave us all a gift. He was released from possibly years of a debilitating disease that would have only gotten worse. We, his family, were given the opportunity to continue living without the absolute sorrow of watching him decline more and more.

However, I will tell you this: it takes fortitude and grit to communicate to medical people what you do and do not want in the way of treatment. Have conversations often with your family, have legal documents supporting what you want, and communicate with your doctors so it is in your medical records. Make sure every member of your family knows what you want. If needed, have multiple conversations with family members to be sure they understand and will honor your wishes.

Earl's request was to have his body donated to the Anatomical Gifts Program at Duke's Medical School. We honored his request. At some point in the future, the medical school will return his ashes to me.

Earl and I had many conversations about what he wanted. He gave his children, and me, clarity: he made saying no to life-extending treatment possible.

> *"Fearlessness is what love seeks . . . such fearlessness exists only in the complete calm that can no longer be shaken by events."* —Hannah Arendt[1]

Speaking of what Earl wanted, we held his Celebration of Life earlier this month. He had requested a dance be held in our church fellowship hall. He didn't care so much about the service. He wanted his friends to have a heck of a good time and dance the night away.

Well, due to Covid protocols, the dancing could not happen. I felt quite sad about that. We did have a lovely Celebration of Life, though. Earl's service was the first gathering the church had offered since it suspended live services during Covid. The minister was generous in offering us the space under the circumstances.

We were limited to a maximum attendance of eighty-two people. Jen posted on her Facebook page that we would live-stream the service, for our relatives and far-away friends who were still not traveling.

Jen and Rich both shared lovely and funny stories. I talked about how my love for Earl deepened during his last years. Earl's friends shared memories, which meant so much to all of us. Earl's nieces and their husbands came from far away, as did two family friends.

We played Harry Chapin's song, "Circle." We hugged and swayed together.

We can make plans for what we hope for when we die. Earl didn't get his dance, but he would have loved his children's remembrances and his friends' stories. It was, all in all, enough.

---

1. Arendt, *Love and Saint Augustine*, 42.

Love,
Juanita

P.S. Author Joyce Rupp, in her book, *Out of the Ordinary*, shares a ritual similar to the one we used to bless Earl's body.[2]

2. Rupp, *Out of the Ordinary: Prayers, Poems, and Reflections for Every Season.*

July 14, 2021

In Kristi Nelson's book, *Wake Up Grateful*, she writes, "Gratefulness helps us embrace the entirety of our experience. It helps you to learn from life as it actually is with nothing left out."[1]

With those words in mind, I want to journal about the experiences I had with my children, grandson, and son-in-law during the later part of Earl's illness.

The trust and vulnerability Earl exhibited with his daughter was beautiful. If Earl was having a visual hallucination, he would ask her about it. "Do you see spiders on the wall?" Jen would look to where her father was pointing, examine the area carefully, and then respond gently, "No, Dad. No spiders here." Earl would nod, trusting her judgment.

The two of them watched episodes of *Star Trek* when she stayed with him, until he found the show too confusing. Then they watched mellower, slower shows. They frequently found something to laugh about together.

She read *Ramona* by Beverly Cleary to her dad, perched on the side of his hospital bed, a role-reversal from when he had read it to her, decades before.

Jen went to an all-night pharmacy, a half hour away, at 1:00 AM to get needed medications for him. On her return, she slept the remainder of the night on the floor, on a yoga mat, next to her dad's bed, so I could rest.

Earl was protective of her. Even in the last week of his life, he requested she not see him at his weakest. Three days before he

---

1. Nelson, *Wake Up Grateful*, 25.

died, he had a meaningful, if somewhat nonlinear, conversation with Jen and her husband about an upcoming "border crossing" he would be making—and that they should be sure to find a good used car for his grandson.

Our son Rich made sure we had ample supplies on his last visit before the pandemic hit. He would check in regularly to see if he could order any supplies for us from his home in Oregon.

When it became clear he would be limited as to how often he could visit due to Covid, Rich initiated FaceTime calls with his dad. I would sit next to Earl and hold the iPad, while Rich took his dad on walking tours of his Oregon environment. Earl relished the connection and the tours.

A week and a half before Earl died, Earl asked me several times a day where Rich was. The hospice nurse suggested Rich get here as soon as possible, if Earl was asking for him. Rich arrived in time to be with his father. He spent the last three nights of his dad's life with him at the hospice residence so the rest of us could try to sleep. Thus, Rich had the privilege of being with his father when his dad died at 4:20 in the early morning.

There was a particularly special moment with our sixteen-year-old grandson and his grandfather. On a day when Earl was unusually confused, he couldn't find the living room while Sam was visiting. I saw the anxiety in Sam's eyes as he watched the confusion. Yet, Sam guided his grandfather to the living room and then, instead of bolting out the door, which would have been understandable, he sat and chatted with his grandfather so I could prepare dinner.

Our son-in-law, Noah, a physician assistant in primary care, patiently answered all of our medical questions—without ever interfering or offering unsolicited advice. One particularly bad night, at around 2:30 AM, Earl fell and I could not pick him up. Noah couldn't pick him up, either. Earl said, "That's okay, all I need is a pillow. I'll sleep on the floor." Noah, who Earl completely trusted, sat on the floor next to Earl and gently talked with him to reassure him that his bed would be more comfortable.

I called 911 for "pick-up assistance" at 3 AM. Noah and Jen stayed with me. Noah watched how the paramedics picked Earl up so he could possibly help Earl the next time—which he successfully did the next morning, when Earl fell again. And it was Noah who first recognized that hospice care was needed and gently conveyed the urgency.

During their 3:00 AM visit, the paramedics suggested they take Earl to the hospital. With no hesitation, I said absolutely not. Earl had been clear with me from the beginning he did not want to spend any time in a hospital. Jen and Noah heard the interchange; they did not interfere. I knew they respected my response and would back me up if need be.

How blessed was our home to have these gentle, caring people assist us in time of need. They were supportive of me and showed such compassion for Earl.

One of the observations my students make, those who take my class entitled, "Insights and Challenges of Parents of Adult Children," is that their adult children criticize their caregiving, giving unsolicited suggestions on how they could do better. Other adult children reverse roles or infantilize their parents, treating their parents like they are children in need of care.

Not once did I feel disrespected by my children. Not once did I feel my family was not supportive. Not once did any of them offer unsolicited advice.

Talk about embracing gratitude! Thank you to my children, grandson, and son-in-law for your trust in me. I believe we were all guided by the spirit of doing the best we could for a man we loved.

The Aftermath: Grief

August 14, 2021

Dear Friends and Family,

I suspect we are all grieving. Covid is making a comeback. The summer that started out hopeful, offering a chance to live more normally, seems to be evaporating. This is a significant loss.

Perhaps the lessons I've learned over the past several months can be helpful to you, too, given the collective grief we are experiencing from Covid.

In grief, I expect to learn many lessons yet unknown.

Here are lessons I have learned so far:

Loneliness or solitude?

In the days and weeks following Earl's death, I felt extraordinarily lonesome. It was hard for me to concentrate on anything. However, I happened to find solace in an old source of comfort: the theologian, Henri Nouwen.

> To live a spiritual life we must first find the courage to enter into the desert of our loneliness and to change it by gentle and persistent efforts into a garden of solitude. The movement from loneliness to solitude, however, is the beginning of any spiritual life because it is the movement from the restless senses to the restful spirit, from

the outward-reaching cravings to the inward-reaching search, from the fearful clinging to the fearless play.[1]

This quote was a magnificent gift; it totally shifted my experience. I recognized that I had been responding to my loneliness with outward-reaching cravings. I was constantly asking myself what I could buy, eat, or watch that would rescue me from my feelings.

Reframing what I was experiencing as solitude, rather than loneliness, stopped my slide. I started writing letters to Earl, something I now enjoy doing almost daily. I began looking for poetry and music I resonated with, to read and listen to. I started to care for my plants with mindfulness. I took a different attitude on my walks, paying attention to what I was seeing and hearing. I began to smile more. I've made friends with solitude.

Getting unstuck.

Before Earl's dementia, I had loved to travel, often by myself, so I was excited to be able to go visit my son in Oregon again. However, as I tried to pack for this first trip since Earl's death, I felt . . . paralyzed. Fear and anxiety swept over me. I hadn't been anywhere since Earl's diagnosis. Could I even do this—step out into the world once again? The thought of leaving the safety of my routines felt overwhelming. For years, my life had been measured by Earl's needs, by the rhythms of his care, and by the rituals that held us steady. Now, my empty suitcase open before me, I felt the weight of both absence and possibility.

I picked up Martha Hickman's book, *Healing After Loss: Daily Meditations for Working Through Grief*, and read:

> It is hard to shake loose of feeling paralyzed. But we can, by starting with just one thing. Baking bread. Visiting a neighbor. Anything to break the logjam. It may seem as fateful as that first "giant step" out of the capsule and into space.[2]

1. Nouwen, *Reaching Out: The Three Movements of Spiritual Life*, 25.
2. Hickman, *Healing After Loss*, 30.

I found I could do one thing. I put my pajamas in the suitcase, then took a break. Later, I packed a second item and walked away. Then, a third item, and so on. The trip was both difficult and wonderful. Now, when I feel paralyzed, I remember I only need to take one step at a time. I do just one thing. And then another.

There is a newborn baby, Nathan, in a home across the street. His parents often sit on their front porch with swaddled Nathan, and wave at neighbors walking by. Their joy is contagious. By doing one small thing—stepping out my front door—I see them. I wave.

With gratitude for life,
Juanita

P.S. My new best friend is a small stuffed rabbit with big floppy ears, who I cuddle with. One of the authors of the many books I have read on caring for someone with dementia wrote that she found comfort in a stuffed teddy bear. I remember wondering, could a stuffie really be helpful? Now, I thank that not-remembered author for the idea. The right stuffed animal does indeed offer comfort. I suspect a beloved pet would offer similar feelings of coziness.

November 1, 2021

Greetings Family and Friends,

When I was in private practice as a grief counselor, I displayed an altar for *Dia de los Muertos* (Day of the Dead) in my waiting room. I hoped it would encourage my clients to become more comfortable talking about death, and to think of ways to honor the memories of their ancestors and loved ones.

I've had a *Dia de los Muertos* altar in my home for many years. I love unwrapping the skeletons and figurines every year and displaying them, along with marigolds, candles, and pictures of loved ones who have died. I give thanks to the wisdom and generosity of the culture of origin of this practice.

May I suggest you take some time to sit quietly and remember your loved ones who have journeyed on?

Love,
Juanita

January 18, 2022

Dear Friends and Family,

One day last month, I slowly reread every card that was sent to Earl and/or me these last few years. I hope every one of you understands my appreciation for your kindnesses in all their forms: cards, plants, mason jars of wildflowers left on our porch, gift cards, financial help, tax prep, chocolate bars, donuts, balloons, birdseed, blankets, desserts, soup, pictures, grocery shopping, transportation, personal services, and your texts and emails. And those who came to see us from miles away. In all these ways and more, we felt your caring and support.

For those of you who came to our home to share stories, and on one occasion play Earl's favorite songs on guitar, you were our shining lights. For those who talked with Earl and helped him feel he mattered, you sustained our belief in loving connection beyond illness. To my family who offered me respite, and all-night help when needed towards the end, you cared with great love.

Thank you, one and all, for making our experience one of thoughtfulness and caring.

Since Earl's death, two experiences have revealed the depth of my grief—both of them connected to medical care. What should have been routine moments instead broke me open, reminding me in an instant what I have lost.

The first was when I had cataract surgeries in October. I was so grateful for my daughter's presence and my son's texts, but oh, how I missed Earl! He would have engaged all the health-care providers with pharmaceutical questions; he would have held my hand while his eyes twinkled with good humor. I was a basket case for a while after the surgeries, so filled with grief. Finally, by writing to Earl and taking long walks, I found my equilibrium again, witnessing the beautiful world my new-and-improved eyes were beholding.

The second experience was a visit to my dentist, to have a crown repaired. Before the dentist started the procedure, I told him my husband had always come with me to these appointments, and how deeply I missed him. As I spoke, my eyes filled with tears. The dentist assured me it was natural to feel my husband's absence. Putting my feelings out in the open left me raw, but also lighter. I was able to proceed with the treatment.

A revelation has come to me in the past few months. While caring for Earl, I was so attuned to his needs, it left little time for me to experience "awe" moments. When I took walks, I was usually focused on how long I was away from home and the need to get back. When we chatted with a friend, I was aware of Earl's level of comfort with the situation, rather than the conversation itself.

The night following Earl's death, I walked outside in the dark for the first time in years. Suddenly, I could go anywhere and for as long as I liked. Gazing at the night sky and stars, listening to the hoot of an owl. I was free; no one needed me. Instead of feeling relieved, I felt so, so sad. That night, I spent hours sitting on the porch, telling Earl about the owl and the stars.

Now however, when I am with others, I can have real conversations without concern. When I walk, I can notice cloud formations, or stop to watch a bunny rabbit, or take in a glorious sunset. The position of my bed often allows me to see the moon in the early morning. I marvel at these experiences. The luxury of breathing deeply, of not being preoccupied, of being wholly present. I can once again experience moments of awe.

Journaling and writing to Earl are my daily practice. When I awake in the morning, I like to listen to a Tara Brach podcast, which often includes meditation.[1] I receive counsel from a hospice social worker. I joyously prepare for my classes and teach remotely. These are my essentials for now.

My friends help me laugh, and have encouraged me to be more comfortable talking on the phone while being together continues to be postponed. My students are enthusiastic learners. My family supports me without complaint.

My friends, feel your human heart, and the goodness for life, Juanita

---

1. *The Tara Brach Podcast,* hosted by Tara Brach.

January 20, 2022

Usually, Duke medical students and staff have an annual ritual at Duke Gardens to honor their "silent partners"—people like Earl, who donated their bodies to the anatomical program. The students and staff write poems and share gratitude. They create paper boats, and set them afloat on the lily pond, in respectful silence.

Ordinarily, families of silent partners are invited to attend this event. Due to Covid protocols, however, no invitations were sent. This was a big loss for Jen and me. However, I did receive a bundle of lovely notes of gratitude from medical students and staff.

Yesterday, the gift coordinator at the Duke anatomical program called to let me know that Earl's remains had been cremated and were ready to be transferred to me.

I had known this call would come—I had been waiting. Yet it still felt like a shock.

The woman on the phone explained that, ordinarily, the exchange of remains is done with "tender care" in Duke Gardens . . . but she had a family emergency and needed to leave town. She gave me a choice: I could wait until she returned to receive the box of Earl's ashes in the gardens, or she could arrange for a very informal "pick up" from a staff member who would meet us in a parking lot.

I loved the idea of a tender exchange in Duke Gardens, but I wanted Earl's ashes to come home as soon as possible. I did not want to wait.

Jen drove. I sat in the passenger seat. As we approached the pick-up location—a loading bay behind a Duke hospital building—for some reason the theme music from *Jaws* ran through my head. The meeting felt rather clandestine!

We pulled into the loading bay. A man was standing beside several Dumpsters, by himself, respectfully holding something the size of a shoebox.

I rolled down my window and waved.

He came over. "Good afternoon, ma'am."

"Hello."

"Your name, please?"

"Juanita Johnson."

He nodded. "Here you go. Be careful. It's heavier than it looks."

The sturdy cardboard box was indeed heavier than it looked. In more ways than one.

Earl Johnson was printed on the top.

The man gave a slight smile, and a nod, then turned and walked away.

And that was that. Earl was coming back home.

March, 24, 2022

It's been almost a year since Earl's death. I am itching to write about my feelings of disappointment and curiosity.

For many years, I counseled all sorts of souls who were grieving, who had lost something dear to them for a variety of reasons: death, divorce, separation, estrangement, miscarriage, violence, diagnosis.

There were often common themes among these people. They felt alone, or misunderstood, or the people they most wanted to support them didn't show up.

I try to be kind and forgiving, so writing this is not easy for me. But the truth is that the family and friends I thought would want to talk with me about the man I loved, do not. They don't acknowledge that Earl existed.

What is wrong with people? Why is it so hard to share sacred space with someone who you care about, by asking about their loved one? Is it because of our discomfort with someone else's pain?

I know there are experts who counsel, "If you want to talk about the person you loved, then you need to initiate the conversation." I can do that—but only if I feel the person I am with is receptive. I seldom feel that someone truly wants to hear what I have to say about my loss.

I will forever be grateful to Connie, who I did not know well, but who sat with me on my living-room couch and started a conversation by saying, "I don't know what I would do if my husband died. How do you do it?" It was an invitation.

I suppose for some, that question might feel intrusive, but I was so eager to share stories of my husband and my own path to finding a new life, I jumped right in. She listened and I talked and talked. What a gift she gave me that day! She was not a close friend, but she was a *bold* friend. I shall always remember her generosity, because that sort of invitation hardly ever happens. She held space for me.

Other extremely meaningful interactions have been with Judy, who, every time we are together, looks me straight in my eyes, and, with sincerity, says, "Tell me how you really are." And then she listens. She, too, holds space for me.

And I'm grateful that my children, son-in-law, and grandson love to talk about Earl. It fills my heart with joy to hear their stories.

I understand people often show their caring with food, flowers, cards, or a book. I know that people show up in different ways. I don't discount their caring. But, at the same time, I, and I suspect billions of others, want a space where we can safely share our stories, so we don't have to pay a grief counselor to listen to us! (If that is even an option.)

Heather Plett writes in *The Art of Holding Space*:

> Holding space is about bearing witness. It's about showing up for a person we care about even when they have nothing to offer in return. It's listening without having to change the narrative or the situation. It's hearing the things in a person's story others overlook.[1]

Let's all get better (yup, me too) at bearing witness with people we care about.

---

1. Plett, *Holding Space*, 2.

May 18, 2022

Dear Friends and Family,

One year ago today, Earl died. Like Rich and Jen do, I have such vivid memories of his last few days. He knew we were with him for his last earthly days with our touches and our voices. My dear one was surrounded with love.

This week, one year later, at my request, Suzanne, my hospice social worker, facilitated a gathering of our family on Zoom. Rich, Jen, Sam, Noah, and I told our favorite stories about dad, grandfather, father-in-law, and husband. We also shared what this past year has been like for us and the many different ways we have grieved.

Our laughter and tears blended together as we reflected on our love for Earl and how we miss him. We ritualized the anniversary with intention and presence. Jen made us each a pillar candle with Earl's picture, for us to light when we miss him. I will take my son's candle to him when I next visit.

This past December, I participated in an online hospice gathering designed to look at ways to cope with the holiday season. One of the suggestions was to give oneself a gift reflective of our loved one. I was intrigued with the possibility of gifting myself something that would offer me comfort, which brings me to give you some background information.

The first summer Earl and I were married, the summer of 1965, we found jobs at a Girl Scout camp in the Ozarks. All the adults who worked there had to have camp names. My name was

Bunny, Earl's was Smiley. For whatever reason, my name stuck. For fifty-four years, Earl affectionately called me Bun or often BR, short for Bunny Rabbit. I have a wall of framed pictures of rabbits Earl drew for me for birthdays and anniversaries.

When I considered what I would like to give myself, I was drawn to investigating ornamental rabbits for my garden. I found a rather whimsical solar rabbit. I gave it to myself, and put it on my back deck. Every night, I am comforted by the white light that radiates from the rabbits' paws. It offers me solace. Before I go to bed, I acknowledge the light and smile.

It truly is remarkable how unpredictable grief is, and how such a small thing as a rabbit holding a solar light can be soothing.

This past year has offered new insights, so many opportunities to mourn, many letters written to Earl, and stories shared. I am blessed with a family who is open to grief. We share our missing of him. We are respectful of the different ways we grieve, and always have each other's backs. I know Earl is not surprised, for he has shown us the way forward.

Warmest wishes,
Juanita

July 15, 2022

Dear Family and Friends,

I'm back with a new update after being encouraged to keep on writing about my experiences with grief and how I'm adapting to a new life.

A few weeks ago, texting back and forth with my son, I wrote:

> I'm thinking about how to have a more interesting life. I have nice friends who I see fairly often. Volunteering at the museum is informative and good for me. I have gotten good at solitude and I try to let it be enough. But I sometimes find myself asking, "Is this all there is?"

The text pretty much describes where I am right now. I'm searching for something more. Do any of you feel that way? I can't thread the needle between grief and Covid. I know Covid plays into my feelings of frustration and loss.

Yes, I understand it's up to me to create a new life for myself. I love teaching, and Zoom has provided the opportunity to connect with students far and wide. Life coaching is rewarding, although coaching on Zoom is different than being eye-to-eye in the same room.

I'm volunteering at the Museum of Durham History, which has proven to be a terrific way for me to meet people. Even so, this business of finding my way as a single person, after being a twosome for fifty-four years, is challenging. It's easy for lonesomeness to creep in.

Here is what saves me when I wonder, "What more is there?" I write to Earl, and every night, I stand at the back door and say good night to the solar light that shines brightly on my deck. These are my private rituals. They help me immensely.

I've been curious how common it is for those who are grieving to find private rituals to be helpful. Can one transcend despair and distress? I read an article that says those who overcome their grief "more quickly" (whatever that means) all had something in common: following the loss, they performed "rituals"—but not typical, public rituals.[1] These rituals were private.

One person returned to the gravesite by themselves once a month. Another cut up and burned all her pictures after a break-up. Another washed her husband's car weekly, as her husband had done prior to his death. A woman whose mom died played "I Miss You Like Crazy" by Natalie Cole, and cried every time she played it.[2]

How do private rituals help? According to research, they help counteract the turbulence and chaos that follows loss.[3] One of the common responses to loss is feeling the world is out of control. Joan Didion wrote in *The Year of Magical Thinking*, "Everything is going along as usual and then all shit breaks loose."[4]

An article in *The Atlantic* said Harvard researchers found that personal rituals "trigger very specific feelings in mourn-ers—the feelings of being in control of their lives."[5] Things are in check. A griever is less likely to feel helpless or powerless. A ritual can offer a connection to the person who has died. This makes sense, don't you think?

The night Joan Didion's husband died of a sudden heart at-tack, she took the money out of his wallet, carefully sorted the bills, opened her wallet and placed his five-dollar bills next to hers, his

1. Norton and Gino, "Rituals Alleviate Grieving," *The Journal of Experimental Psychology*.

2. Norton and Gino, "Rituals Alleviate Grieving," *The Journal of Experimental Psychology*.

3. Norton and Gino, "Rituals Alleviate Grieving," *The Journal of Experimental Psychology*.

4. Didion, *Magical Thinking*, 3.

5. Smith, "In Grief, Try Personal Rituals," *The Atlantic*.

ten-dollar bills next to hers, and so on. Didion writes that her husband would have approved. She was showing him, and herself, she could cope and would survive.

> "*Grief turns out to be a place none of us know until we reach it.*" —Joan Didion, *The Year of Magical Thinking.*[6]

When I write to Earl, he sometimes responds in my mind's eye. Recently, he reminded me I am in transition. I'm experiencing the chaos and uncertainty of the "Neutral Zone," a term coined by researcher and author William Bridges.[7] This is the time between the old reality and identity, and the new. So, I'm creating new processes, learning about what has yet to emerge. This is a time I need to breathe and trust the process . . . and not be impatient.

In *Bomb Shelter: Love, Time, and Other Explosives*, author Mary Laura Philpott writes:

> No one knows how anything is going to turn out, which means you can't get all indignant because it turned out differently. There's only the way it turns out. There's only the ending that was always going to happen, you just didn't know it yet.[8]

Take care y'all. Love well.

Warmly,
Juanita

---

6. Didion, *Magical Thinking*, 188.
7. Bridges, *Transitions: Making Sense of Life Changes*.
8. Philpott, *Bomb Shelter*, 238.

April 7, 2023

Dear Friends and Family,

It's spring in North Carolina. The wrens have made a nest in my daughter's mailbox next door. Cardinals have nested in her porch light. I have two sets of wrens' nests in unused flower pots. What a joy to hear their little chirps. I hope spring has sprung where you live, with blue skies and some warmth.

> *"We do not comprehend ruins until we ourselves are in ruin."*
> —Heinrich Heine[1]

In the early days after Earl died, a phone call from my cousin would inevitably include a conversation about what books he had been reading. I loved hearing what had caught his interest. He mentioned *Suzanne and Gertrude*.[2] My cousin thought I might like it. At the time, I couldn't read anything. My brain was too scrambled and grief-stricken. I doubted I could read an entire book, but I was very intrigued by how my cousin described the story. The book jacket description:

> Suzanne has arranged her life to suit her solitariness, living quietly on her untended hill farm. Her days are a word-shy negotiation, caught between indifference and uncertainty. Into this world comes Gertrude, a wandering donkey. Together they form an unlikely alliance; each protecting the solitude of the other. It's a tale of intermittent griefs and wonderments. How do we live,

1. quoted in Lang, *Chaos and Cosmos*, 41.
2. Nichols, *Suzanne and Gertrude: A Novel*.

not just with each other, but with memories, with imper-
manence, with the inevitable melancholy of being?[3]

I did read the book. In fact, over the course of the last two years, I
have read it three times. The story has had a deep-rooted impact
on me.

My experience of having Earl die, and adjusting to caring
for myself, has resulted in feelings similar to what Suzanne felt:
"The day, towards evening . . . becomes tomblike. Not a whisper,
no murmur."[4] And although a donkey did not appear in my life
(thank goodness!) a few friends, my children, my son-in-law, and
my grandson, have given me the love and connection equivalent
to—or better than—what the donkey offered Suzanne.

Still, I miss my companion of fifty-four years so much that
I ache. Especially when I've read a good book and want to share
it with him. Or watch a British mystery and know how much he
would enjoy sitting next to me as we viewed the program together.
Meditating on the deck with a chorus of birds in the background,
taking long walks, sharing memories. Earl anchored me.

I think about when I first felt that anchor. We had been dating several months, and we were on one of our afternoon campus
walks. Earl invited me to look up. Above us was a large bird, soar-
ing in the brilliant, cloudless, blue sky. With awe in his voice, Earl
told me it was a red-tailed hawk. He told me that these hawks flap
their wings in a rhythmic pattern, to gain lift and propel themselves through the air. He saw the magnificence of something I
had never even noticed. I fell in love with him that afternoon.
The experience of seeing the world in new ways, through his
eyes—I never wanted it to end.

It will soon be two years since Earl died. Grandson Sam and
I have planted native shrubs, Earl's favorites. My Durham family
and I are having dinner, a get-together to tell Earl stories. I will

3. Nichols, *Suzanne and Gertrude*, jacket.
4. Nichols, *Suzanne and Gertrude*, 39.

be in Oregon on Earl's death day, May eighteenth. Rich and I will make a tiny altar on our table at a special restaurant.

I find naming what I've learned helpful, so here goes:

- A stuffed animal is an indispensable sleeping companion.
- The habits Earl and I established to keep him on an even keel continue to serve me well.
- When I was ready, counseling sessions with a hospice social worker (available to any family, for up to thirteen months following the death of a loved one) were times I always looked forward to.
- Keeping a journal, and writing letters to Earl, has kept his spirit close.
- Finding a good match for a place to volunteer and engage with new people has been incredibly helpful. (Thank you to Maurita, who suggested the museum.)
- Cultivating new friendships has lightened my spirit.
- Seeking out people who can tell me stories about Earl makes me laugh and cry (a special thanks to my children).
- I'm eternally grateful for the very few friends who look me in the eye and ask me how I really am.
- I have been greatly changed by my new reality. I will not "recover." I will not "move on." One does not return to normal. Staying true to myself, holding fiercely to my own heart, my core, this is what guides me.
- I find that survival in grief lies in finding the connection between the life I had and the life that has been thrust upon me.

On another note. I am privileged to teach classes on death and dying, autobiographies, and writing ethical wills. The participants in my most recent "Living with Intention—Dying Prepared" class asked if we could continue meeting monthly. We call our ongoing monthly meetings "Living-Dying." Talking about living well and dying with intention, as a group, has changed how we live. Those of us in the circle are finding that our lives become more meaningful by having life's most important conversations. When we are open to a life of endings, it helps us live more fully in the present. Our deliberate time together offers us an expanded awareness of how facing mortality can open us to gratitude, connection, and what matters most.

> *"Death walks with us through our entire life. The best thing I can suggest is that we all get better acquainted with our constant companion."* —Michael Hebb[5]

Thank you for reading this update. I hope it will help you walk your own beautiful path with intention.

Love,
Juanita

P.S. By far the best book on grief I've read is *It's Okay That You're Not Okay*.[6]

---

5. Hebb, *Let's Talk about Death*, 14.

6. Devine, *It's Okay That You're Not Okay: Meeting Grief and Loss in a Culture that Doesn't Understand*.

August 17, 2023

Greetings All,

It has been quite a summer of terrible fires, rains, and heat. I hope you are okay where you live.

My city was hit with a quick, out-of-nowhere storm. The wind and torrential rain tore huge trees from their roots and left my part of the city without power for three days and nights.

In May, the second anniversary of Earl's dying day provided me and my family with lovely rituals. Before I explain the rituals we found meaningful, I want to encourage you to consider expanding on the ritual-making in your own life.

Often birthdays are celebrated using a yearly ritual, which may be passed on in families. The rituals surrounding when a loved one dies are also important. But too often in our busy culture, we ignore the opportunity to enhance a meaningful occasion with a ritual.

Rituals can calm anxieties, help us find deeper meaning, and invite community. A ritual, when done well, allows individuals to be vulnerable, fully present, and engaged.

I know a family who spent a week together as an extended family after the worst of the pandemic was over. They renewed relationships and shared their Covid stories with one another. At the end of the week, the entire extended family gathered outdoors. Everyone was invited to find a rock or stone. As each person placed their stone in the middle of the circle, they said a sentence or two about what the week had meant to them. It was a beautiful and meaningful way for them to say goodbye.

To acknowledge Earl's second dying-day anniversary, I had the opportunity to participate in two very different but incredibly meaningful rituals.

Following a meal with my daughter, son-in-law, and grandson, I read entries from Earl's 1962 journal, where he described his undergraduate college years. He wrote about the books he read. (Jen looked up the titles. It was great fun for us to imagine him enjoying pulp science-fiction books of the 1960's.) Earl wrote about the movies he had seen and the two young women he was dating. Together we laughed—and shed a few tears—as we read about his undergraduate college years.

Another anniversary ritual was with my son in Oregon. We went to a special restaurant for dinner. Rich wore a shirt of his dad's. Together we created a small altar on the table, which included a beautiful marble that Rich had a glass artist make for me. Inside the marble were a few of Earl's ashes. We told stories of remembrance and ate wonderful food. We were seated by a window, and as we ate, the sky filled with heat lightning. It was magical. We both felt Earl's presence.

Rituals, done well, provide us with meaning and sometimes an ache in our heart. Rituals help us feel our full range of human emotions. They give us the opportunity to celebrate all the messiness of life.

I wish you well,
Juanita

November 9, 2023

Dear Friends and Family,

It's been a while. I trust you are taking care of yourselves. We are all settling into the early darkness of late fall. Perhaps that allows you to slow your pace a bit? Time to take a deep breath.

My "new" life continues to emerge.

Earl especially enjoyed Fridays. He loved to listen to weekly news shows on NPR. As Earl's ability to assess reality changed, he often became irritable and unpleasant after listening to the recap of the weekly news on the radio (something many people experience, right?). It took me a while to see the connection between the news and his irritation. My goal was to keep Earl at peace and not deliberately do anything that caused distress. It was time to change the Friday routine. I had to fib, something caregivers become skilled at when living with someone with dementia. I told Earl that his favorite shows had gone off the air. I suggested we listen to music at that time instead. That became our new routine. I found I enjoyed the respite from news, too. I stuck with this change.

Recently *The Good Life Project* podcast invited listeners to send an audio recording describing their daily habits.[1] I recorded the five habits that have changed my life. My audio recording went like this:

> When my husband was diagnosed with a cognitive disease, it became apparent some of our habits would need

1. "Five Life-Changing Habits," *The Good Life Project*, September 15, 2022.

to change in order for our home to remain tranquil. After my husband died, I have kept the changes we made. They have profoundly influenced my life.

My five habits:

1. I only read the news. I don't watch television or video news. I do not listen to news on the radio.

2. After supper, I connect with nature. If it is light outside, I take a walk. If it is dark, I walk onto my deck and listen to the early sounds of the night and look at the sky.

3. I turn the TV off at 8:00 PM, even if I'm in the middle of watching a show. No exceptions.

4. Journaling, jigsaw puzzles, an audio book, reading, or music, are how I spend my time from 8:00 PM until bedtime.

5. When I'm tucked into bed, I often end my day with meditation.

If it hadn't become necessary to change our routine to eliminate news from my husband's options, I may never have found the peacefulness that now surrounds me with these five habits.

Another part of my "new" life is the weekly volunteer time I spend at the Museum of Durham History. I encounter people from different parts of Durham, as well as from all over the world. This week at the museum, a man in his early fifties came in. He said he is an electrical engineer; he takes care of electrical problems for the Amtrak station across the street, and several other buildings that are close to the museum. He loves history and was excited to see pictures of the buildings he cares for from earlier times. As we chatted, he told me his mother recently died and he doesn't know how he and his brothers will get through Thanksgiving dinner without her. I shared with him our custom of placing a candle where Earl used to sit, and leaving his chair empty. The man was thrilled with the suggestion. He thought his brothers would like it, too.

"It would be a way to honor our mother, who always sat at the head of the table," he said.

My heart swelled. A random connection. A meaningful conversation.

That's it for now. Thanks for reading this.

Treat yourself with kindness,
Juanita

May 1, 2024

Greetings to You,

How many of you remember May Day baskets? My mother filled small, handmade construction-paper baskets with tiny purple violets from our yard. We would hang these baskets on our neighbors' doorknobs. Such an endearing ritual, now long gone.

As part of my volunteer gig at the Museum of Durham History, I train volunteers on how to interview, and audio record, the histories of people from Durham.

At Duke University, there is a program that centers Black storytelling. The museum and the Black storytelling center are considering a joint project, recording audio histories of long-time Durham residents. Recently, I consulted with one of the coordinators of the Duke program. As the two of us chatted, she mentioned that her husband had been drafted after receiving an advanced degree in engineering and working for IBM in Atlanta. Her husband was stationed at Fort Myer in Washington, D.C. and was assigned to the Pentagon.

I asked her what years her husband was at the Pentagon—it turns out our husbands were there at the same time! They even worked on the same floor. Did they ever have the occasion to meet? We'll never know.

It was grand fun for the two of us to share our experiences living in the D.C. area from 1967–1969, a time when there was so much upheaval in the world and in our country. The two of us realized we had both participated in a demonstration in front of the

White House in support of Eartha Kitt's vocal denunciation of the Vietnam War on January 19, 1968. We both had stories to tell about how much our participation in that action impacted us.

This sharing was an opportunity to recall the early years of my marriage. Remembering the special friends Earl and I met while we lived in D.C. The tiny apartment we rented. The fires in the nighttime sky over D.C. during the uprisings after the assassination of Dr. Martin Luther King, Jr.

All those memories came flooding back. In my mind's eye, I was there. I could see Earl, hear his voice telling me about his work. I could hear myself sharing with him stories of the commute to my job, and the people I met. Earl and I talked about the fun picnics we had in parks with his army friends. Our attempts to bake bread. The cockroaches in the kitchen. And the laughter, oh the laughter . . . and the profound gratitude we felt that his post was stateside.

If you have experienced the death of someone you love, you understand the mix of both sorrow and joy when you have the opportunity to reminisce.

When someone says to me, "I don't want to upset you by talking about Earl," my response is always, "Earl is in my heart every day. Talking about him is a gift you can give me."

Although friends and family have been generous and kind to me, what warms my heart and brings tears to my eyes, is when an email or text arrives with a message of remembrance about Earl. Or when I see someone at the market who looks me in the eye and says, "I remember when Earl . . . "

Earl's third dying-day anniversary is May eighteenth. I will be sharing Earl stories with my family in Durham and in Oregon. As a family, we relish remembering.

Stories connect us and enhance our love for one another. My friends, we are all storytellers. When you are with someone who has had a loved one die, ask them to tell you a story about their person. Or tell them a story of your time with that individual. If you send a card, include a memory or story of the person who has died.

We are vulnerable, authentic humans when we listen to each other's stories.

Love,
Juanita

October 17, 2024

Earl and I met and began dating while I attended Stephens College and he was a student at Mizzou (University of Missouri) in Columbia. We attended a Methodist church on Sunday mornings. We seldom saw people in their twenties there. It suited us though, because growing up, we had both spent Sunday mornings in church with our families.

We married and began our life together in Colorado (after summer jobs at a camp in the Ozarks), where I took classes, and Earl pursued a Ph.D. at Colorado State University in Fort Collins. One of the first things we did, which became a life-long habit for us, was to find a church that suited our liberal-progressive lifestyle. Wherever we lived, our radar was alert to find a church that offered small groups as well as a nurturing, inclusive Sunday experience.

With only a few exceptions, we have always found our best friends in the small church groups we attended and enjoyed so very much. It was the small group in Colorado that supported us when Earl was drafted. When we moved to Fredericksburg, Virginia, we participated in a couples group at an Episcopal church we loved. We read *I'm Okay You're Okay* and laughed ourselves silly during discussions and reflections.[1]

When we moved to Norwich, a small town in upstate New York, Earl and I facilitated a discussion group within a (relatively) liberal United Methodist church for fifteen years. We studied many topics, and best of all, we supported one another through our ups and downs. We led Marriage Enrichment groups in our home. We both loved being hospitable.

1. Harris, *I'm Okay You're Okay*.

Our fourth move, which would be our last, was to Durham, North Carolina, to be near our grandson and his mom and dad. As was our usual custom, we found a liberal-progressive congregation. This time it was a Unitarian-Universalist church fellowship, which provided small groups that grounded us. We had been active in this spiritual community for sixteen years when Earl was diagnosed. I had served on the church board and led several small groups. Earl was deeply involved in the small group that studied *A Course in Miracles* (ACIM), which met at the fellowship.[2] The ACIM group meant so much to Earl. I'm grateful that its group members continued to support and care about him after his diagnosis.

When Earl was diagnosed with Lewy body dementia, I informed the fellowship leadership team—and then found myself confused and frustrated by the lack of communication or follow-up from fellowship friends or clergy.

My entire life, I had been able to count on my church family to offer comfort and support when needed. Thus, the lack of even an occasional text message or email from church leadership—anything to acknowledge we were being thought of or inquire how we were—was extraordinarily confusing to me. Yes, there were a few people on the "care team" who contacted us. Which was appreciated. But I felt I had been abandoned. It hurt.

After Earl died, I was able to communicate to a person in leadership my disappointment that I hadn't been cared for. They acknowledged that yes, that had happened.

I decided to return to the fellowship a few months after Earl died. My daughter went with me for a few weeks, and then I went alone, and sat alone. No one in the congregation offered to sit with me. One Sunday, a medical professional who had treated Earl, sat across from me. He never made eye contact or spoke to me, nor did any of my friends as I left the service.

Covid protocols had ended, yet there was a lingering hesitation from some to engage. I understood that. I also understood that this fellowship was much larger than other churches we had

2. Schucman, *A Course in Miracles*.

been a part of. There were more people to support. I was quite generous in my rationales as to why I wasn't acknowledged. Yet, I felt sadder and more adrift attending Sunday services than any other time of the week.

As a way of coping with my confusion and hurt, I wrote to Earl, which always calmed me. When I finished writing, I knew I needed to find a different, more fulfilling way to find comfort in my spiritual life. Thus, I began investing in poet David Whyte's online "Three Sunday Series."[3] His poetry, his voice, and wise words, soothed me for a year and a half.

And then, I felt a shift inside. More forgiving, more looking forward instead of back. I wanted to return to my Unitarian fellowship to see how it felt.

A year and three-quarters after walking away, I walked back in.

It felt brave to return. And I'm glad I did.

> *"Courage is the measure of our heartfelt participation with life, with another, with community."* —David Whyte[4]

3. Whyte, "Three Sunday Series."
4. Whyte, *Consolations*, 51.

November 14, 2024

Dear Friends and Family,

Occasionally, I teach a class on writing an ethical will. An ethical will is a letter that conveys your values, experiences, and life lessons to your loved ones.[1] My inspiration for teaching the class are the letters my dad began writing to me when I was fourteen. He wrote to me periodically until his death when I was twenty-three. His uplifting letters have helped me through many dark nights of the soul. To have his love for me demonstrated in his letters has always provided a soothing balm.

In the first letter my dad wrote, he described how he felt holding me for the first time. He shared his worries for his beloved wife who had had a difficult time giving birth. He wrote about putting up a Christmas tree in our home on that snowy December day to occupy himself while he was restless, excited, and needed something to do. What a treasure his letters are!

Earl wrote two ethical wills to his children. The first he wrote decades ago, the other more recently, to be given to them upon his death. His writings conveyed his love for them, and his desire for them to live their own unique lives. The letters were short, to the point, and reflected Earl's values beautifully. He gave his children an everlasting gift.

When my excited daughter called home in April of 2004 to share the news that she and Noah were going to be parents, I knew

1. Baines, *Ethical Wills* and Papritz, *Legacy Letters.*

I would celebrate the welcomed news by starting a journal for my November-arriving grandchild.

My goal was to record my grandchild's life up until his graduation from high school. The writing also allowed me an avenue to sprinkle in some grandmotherly wisdom. I gave my grandson the completed journal for his graduation. Eighteen years of good times, scary times, quotes, poetry, and love, poured into the pages.

I hope Sam will keep the journal and occasionally reread parts of it when he has his own dark nights of the soul.

In one of my classes, a student stated they hoped they didn't die suddenly because they wanted the opportunity to tell their loved ones how they felt about them one last time. We have no guarantees how our life will end. We can, however, write to our loved ones now. We might write about how much they mean to us, and how they enrich our life, and give them our blessing.

The key to ethical wills, legacy letters, whatever you call them, is to share what you value, what you have experienced, and life lessons. The letter can be placed in an envelope, with a name on it, and put with important papers. I urge you to do this while you can.

Thinking through what is truly important to you is a way to become more fully alive, intentional, and vibrant, even while facing the fact that life does change and eventually ends. Sharing with loved ones in a thoughtful and reflective way is very satisfying. You have the opportunity to give those you care for a tangible, invaluable, lasting gift. Something precious for them to read and reread when they have their own dark night of the soul.

Warmly,
Juanita

April 14, 2025

Happy Spring to One and All,

On the eighteenth of May, it will be four years since Earl's death. As is true for anyone who has experienced a significant loss, my path has had many twists and turns.

Recently, one of my students said she was "bathing in the stillness" of her life. I exclaimed, "Yes!" when she said those words, as they resonate with what I have found as well.

In *Drinking from the River of Light*, Mark Nepo writes beautifully about how introspection opens a more meaningful embrace of reality: "The goal is not to get dirty or stay clean, but to stay as alive as possible by meeting experience and staying clear."[1] I love his use of a window as metaphor.

Nepo says that love, honesty, and expression are what clear the window of the heart.[2] The more we inhabit love, honesty, and expression, the more we clear and thin the window between in-here and out-there. This thinning between the inner world and the outer world brings us closer to our true life.

Thanks to an insightful therapist who has dragged me deeper into my inner life, I have become content. I know this, because I can laugh with gusto again! Truly, this is a benchmark for me. Where once looking out the window often looked gray, now I see sunlight.

1. Nepo, *Drinking from the River of Light: The Life of Expression*, 76.
2. Nepo, *Drinking from the Rivier of Light*.

Earl's spiritual journey extended over decades. I was the beneficiary of his insights; many rubbed off on me. When Earl was dying, we talked about what life would be like for me without him by my side. I can hear Earl say, "Look out the window, you will find a way forward there."

To honor Earl is to keep choosing life, to keep seeking beauty, to let joy find me when it can.

The loss hasn't changed, but I have.

Onward,
Juanita

P.S. Using my years of updates and journal notes, I am writing the story of my last years with Earl, and my pathway with grief. I have no idea if it will ever be published, but I am having a wonderful time writing it. Thank you to those of you who have encouraged me to collate these notes, write, and reflect.

Epilogue

During our fifty-four years of marriage, my husband Earl and I built a life woven with love, laughter, and shared memories. But when Lewy body dementia began to unravel that tapestry, I found myself navigating a new role—not just as his wife, but as his care partner, witness, and advocate.

I wrote the following, three and half years after he died, to explore the profound shifts in our relationship: the quiet heartbreaks, the unexpected joys, and most of all, the enduring power of love.

Love in the Time of Forgetting

Diagnosis: Lewy body dementia

Conversations

Let there be no suffering by either of us

Never questioned I would be with him

Not a caregiver—a partner

He is kind

I am patient

Lying on the couch together—rubbing my feet until he falls asleep

He says the sun is the "kitty-cat sun"

The front porch is our sanctuary—bird songs, waves, and hellos

Slicing oranges into bite size pieces

Listening to Peter, Paul, and Mary and the Kingston Trio

Dancing together in the kitchen

Reading letters he wrote to me out loud

Holding hands and talking about dying

My beloved says he is ready to die but not to leave me

Tears glisten in both of our eyes

Love ripens—knowing our time is fleeting

The bedroom becomes a hospital room

Orange paint spots on clothes—designate front from back

Bed tray—his new favorite thing—asks for breakfast in bed

Sleeping hours and hours—

never knowing when he might wake up—or how I'm to fill the time

Nighttime stories—every night

Meditation—breathing in breathing out

Nighttime ritual, "I'll see you in the morning light"

Medicine makes him randy—reduce dosage—no brainer

Feces on the floor—so what, just pick it up

Babies on the front porch—politely ask their mommas to take them home

Spiders on the walls—a broom eliminates them

He grabs my hair and pulls

Wraps heavy leg over me and traps me

Pushes me out of bed

It's the REM sleep—never done on purpose

Time to sleep in separate beds

Yet we join for 4 AM snuggles—

immediately drifting off to sleep with arms wrapped around each other

Speaking truth—sometimes hurtful

Spending so much time alone while he sleeps

Watching a brilliant mind shrink

No sense of injustice . . . just acceptance

Not a caregiver

This is a partnership

I never lose my sense of self

Small moments of smiles—especially when grandson, our children, or son-in-law visit

Laughter has faded—didn't realize how much I miss it

Body falling too often—alert to an infection—treat the infection or let the body fail?

Easy decision because of the many conversations we have had

No to the hospital at 3 AM

Peace, dignity, simplicity, love, the breath

You don't keep someone alive because you don't want to be alone

Wholly present in the now—that's all there is

Embracing his dying

His daughter, who brings fresh baby roses to his room

His last words to me: "I am ready to leave"

His son speaks the last goodbye

The three of us touch his now-still body—reciting a prayer

I remember the small rituals—

The conversations

Dancing in the kitchen

Slicing oranges into tiny pieces

Lying on the couch in the sunlight

Watching the birds from the front porch

Siting together holding hands

The nightly reading

And breathing in and breathing out

I open up the front door, step outside into the warm spring night air.

The first time I've been outdoors at night in four years.

The night sky is filled with twinkling stars, a half moon, and, oh my—

I hear an owl, which makes my heart sing.

I am free to go wherever I please.

I find myself sitting in my chair on the porch, next to his empty one.

I describe what I can see, and what I am experiencing,

to the sweet man who accepted a diagnosis with dignity,

and made the best of the time he had left.

And I whisper to him,

"I'll see you in the morning light."

Bibliography

A Network of Grateful Living. *Everyday Gratitude: Inspiration For Living Life as a Gift.* Adams, MA: Storey, 2018.

Albom, Mitch. *Tuesdays with Morrie.* New York: Crown, 2007.

Arendt, Hannah. *Love and Saint Augustine.* Chicago: University of Chicago Press, 1996.

Aurelius, Marcus. *The Meditations of Marcus Aurelius.* Boulder, CO: Shambhala, 2019.

Baines, Barry. *Ethical Wills: Putting Your Values on Paper.* New York: Hachette, 2006.

Benjamin, Melanie. *The Children's Blizzard.* New York: Random House, 2021.

Boss, Pauline. *Ambiguous Loss: Learning to Live with Unresolved Grief.* Cambridge, MA: Harvard University Press, 2000.

Bridges, William. *Transitions: Making Sense of Life Changes.* New York: Balance, 2019.

Chapin, Harry. *Sniper and Other Love Songs.* New York: Elektra, 1972. LP.

Chapman, Gary et al. *Keeping Love Alive as Memories Fade: The Five Love Languages and the Alzheimer's Journey.* Chicago: Northfield, 2016.

———. *The Five Love Languages: How to Express Heartfelt Commitment to Your Mate.* United States: Moody, 2009.

Chittister, Joan and Rowan Williams. *Uncommon Gratitude: Alleluia for All That Is.* Collegeville, MN: Liturgical Press, 2010.

Chodron, Pema. *The Wisdom of No Escape: And the Path of Loving-Kindness.* London: Shambhala Publications, 2010.

Clearly, Beverly. *Ramona.* New York: Harper Collins, 1984.

Devine, Megan. *It's Okay That You're Not Okay: Meeting Grief and Loss in a Culture That Doesn't Understand.* Louisville, CO: Sounds True, 2017.

Didion, Joan. *The Year of Magical Thinking.* New York: Alfred A. Knopf, 2005.

DuBose, Julie. *Effortless Beauty: Photography As an Expression of Eye, Mind, and Heart.* Halifax, Nova Scotia: Milksang, 2013.

"Five Life-Changing Habits." Hosted by Jonathan Fields. *The Good Life Project.* September 15, 2022. https://www.goodlifeproject.com/podcast/the-big-5-life-changing-habits-jonathan-fields.

Fronsdal, Gil. *The Issue at Hand: Essays on Buddhist Mindfulness Practice.* Morocco: Bookland, 2008.

Gibran, Kahil. *The Prophet.* New York: Knopf, 1923.

Gulley, Philip. *Hometown Tales: Reflections of Kindness, Peace, and Joy.* San Francisco: Harper One, 2007.

Hanh, Thich Nhat. *Call Me by my True Names: The Collected Poems of Thich Nhat Hanh.* Berkeley, CA: Parallax, 2022.

———. *Living Buddha, Living Christ.* New York: Riverhead, 2007.

Harris, Thomas. *I'm Okay You're Okay.* New York: Harper & Row, 1967.

Hebb, Michael. *Let's Talk about Death (over Dinner): An Invitation and Guide to Life's Most Important Conversation.* United States: Grand Central, 2018.

Hickman, Martha Whitmore. *Healing After Loss: Daily Meditations for Working Through Grief.* New York: William Morrow, 1994.

Hoblitzelle, Olivia Ames. *Ten Thousand Joys and Ten Thousand Sorrows: A Couple's Journey Through Alzheimer's.* New York: Tarcher, 2010.

Johnson, Robert A. *We: Understanding the Psychology of Romantic Love.* San Francisco: Harper One, 2009.

Kelly, Scott. "I Spent a Year in Space and Have Tips on Isolation." *The New York Times* (March 3, 2020). https://www.nytimes.com/2020/03/21/opinion/scott-kelly-coronavirus-isolation.html.

Lang, Karen. *Chaos and Cosmos: On the Image in Aesthetics and Art History.* Ithaca, NY: Cornell University Press, 2006.

Lewy Body Dementia Association. "Symptoms." *Lbda.org.* https://www.lbda.org/symptoms.

Lewy Body Society, The. "Symptoms." *Lewybody.org.* https://www.lewybody.org/information-and-support/symptoms.

Limelighters, The. *Joy Across the Land.* Hollywood: GNP Crescendo, 1993. CD.

McConaughey, Matthew. *Greenlights.* New York: Random House, 2020.

McDonald, Helen. *Vesper Flights.* New York: Grove, 2020.

———. *H is for Hawk.* New York: Grove, 2015.

"Metta Meditation: A Complete Guide to Loving-Kindness." *Lion's Roar: Buddhist Wisdom for Our Time.* https://www.lionsroar.com/metta-meditation-guide.

Nelson, Kristi. *Wake Up Grateful: The Transformative Practice of Taking Nothing for Granted.* North Adams, MA: Storey, 2020.

Nepo, Mark. *Drinking from the River of Light: The Life of Expression.* Louisville, CO: Sounds True, 2019.

Neshama, Rivvy. *Recipes for a Sacred Life: True Stories and a Few Miracles.* England: Divine Arts, 2013.

Neupert, Shevaun D., Claire M. Growney, Xianghe Zhu, Julia K. Sorensen, Emily L. Smith, and Jan Hannig. "BFF: Bayesian, Fiducial, and Frequentist

Analysis of Cognitive Engagement among Cognitively Impaired Older Adults." *Entropy* 23, no. 4 (2021) 428. https://doi.org/10.3390/e23040428

Nichols, Jeb Loy. *Suzanne and Gertrude: A Novel.* United States: WW Norton, 2019.

Norris, Gunilla. *Being Home: Discovering the Spiritual in the Everyday.* Santa Monica, CA: Hidden Spring, 2002.

Norton, Michael I., and Francesca Gino. "Rituals Alleviate Grieving for Loved Ones, Lovers, and Lotteries." *Journal of Experimental Psychology: General* 143 (2014) 266–72. https://doi.org/10.1037/a0031772.

Nouwen, Henri J. M. *Reaching Out: The Three Movements of the Spiritual Life.* New York: Doubleday, 1975.

Ostaseski, Frank. *The Five Invitations: Discovering What Death Can Teach Us About Living Fully.* New York: Flatiron, 2019.

Papritz, Carley. *The Legacy Letters: His Wife, His Children, His Final Gift.* Mayfield, MA: King's, 2014.

Pascal, Blaise. *Pensées.* Translated by A. J. Krailsheimer. New York: Penguin Classics, 1995.

Pennebaker, James and Joshua Smyth. *Opening Up by Writing It Down.* New York: Guilford, 2016.

Philpott, Mary Laura. *Bomb Shelter: Love, Time, and Other Explosives.* New York: Atria, 2022.

Plett, Heather. *The Art of Holding Space: A Practice of Love, Liberations, and Leadership.* United States: Page Two Books, 2020.

Rademakers, Jan. *World Hits on Harmonica.* Australia: Axis, 1980. LP.

Rainer, Jackson. "How Grief Changes Two Years after a Loss: Moving Forward While Learning Lessons about Grief and Living with the Loss." *Next Avenue* (November 12, 2018). https://www.nextavenue.org/second-year-after-loved-ones-death.

"Repairing Our Hearts." Hosted by Tara Brach. *The Tara Brach Podcast.* December 30, 2020. https://www.tarabrach.com/repairing-hearts-rain-compassion.

Robin's Wish. Directed by Tyler Norwood. Los Angeles: Quotable Pictures, 2020.

Rohr, Richard. *Falling Upward: A Spirituality for the Two Halves of Life.* Hoboken, NJ: Jossey-Bass, 2023.

———. *The Wisdom Pattern: Order, Disorder, Reorder.* Cincinnati, OH: Franciscan Media, 2020.

Roosevelt, Eleanor. *You Learn by Living.* Louisville, KY: Westminster John Knox, 1983.

Rupp, Joyce. *Out of the Ordinary: Prayers, Poems, and Reflections for Every Season.* Notre Dame, IN: Ava Maria, 2011.

Schucman, Helen. *A Course in Miracles.* New York: The Foundation for Inner Peace, 2007.

Sedaris, David. *Calypso.* New York: Hachette, 2018.

Slaght, Jonathan. *Owls of the Eastern Ice: A Quest to Find and Save the World's Largest Owl.* New York: Farrah, Straus, Giroux, 2020.

Smith, Emily Esfahani. "In Grief, Try Personal Rituals." *The Atlantic* (March 14, 2014). https://www.theatlantic.com/health/archive/2014/03/in-grief-try-personal-rituals/284397.

Snyder, Pat. *Treasures in the Darkness: Extending the Early Stage of Lewy Body Dementia, Alzheimer's, and Parkinson's Disease.* United States: Create Space, 2012.

Whiteman, Honor. "Lewy Body Dementia: Unrecognized and Misdiagnosed." *Medical News Today* (November 6, 2015). https://www.medicalnewstoday.com/articles/302230.

Whyte, David. "Three Sundays Series." *David Whyte.* https://davidwhyte.com/three-sundays-overview.

———. *Consolations: The Solace, Nourishment, and Underlying Meaning of Everyday Words.* Langley, WA: Many Rivers, 2021.

Wood, Douglas. *Old Turtle.* Duluth, MN: Pfeifer-Hamilton, 1992.

Author's Note: The Lewy Body Dementia Association (LBDA) is the leading national organization dedicated to improving the lives of LBD families by raising awareness, providing support and educational resources, and advancing research. Find them at https://lbda.org.